Patellar Instability Surgery
in Clinical Practice

Vicente Sanchis-Alfonso
Editor

Patellar Instability Surgery in Clinical Practice

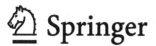 Springer

Editor
Vicente Sanchis-Alfonso
Depto. Cirugia Ortopédica
Hospital Arnau de Vilanova
Valencia
Spain

Originally published as part of Anterior Knee Pain and Patellar Instability, 2nd Ed (ISBN: 978-0-85729-506-4) in 2011

ISBN 978-1-4471-4500-4   ISBN 978-1-4471-4501-1   (eBook)
DOI 10.1007/978-1-4471-4501-1
Springer London Heidelberg New York Dordrecht

Library of Congress Control Number: 2012953482

Printed on acid-free paper

Springer is part of Springer Science+Business Media (www.springer.com)

Preface

Among all the extensor mechanism pathologies, lateral patellar instability is of great interest not only for the general orthopedic surgeon, but also for the knee specialist. The procedure that is most frequently performed to treat lateral patellar instability is the medial patellofemoral ligament (MPFL) reconstruction. The reason for this great interest in this procedure is obvious. Medial patellofemoral ligament reconstruction is the most frequently performed procedure in the extensor mechanism. It also is the most predictable and has the best clinical results of all the procedures in the extensor mechanism. This is the reason why we have decided to publish this small book as a spin-off of the original book *Anterior Knee Pain and Patellar Instability*. In this monograph, we analyze the different reconstruction techniques, step by step, for the MPFL reconstruction, as well as other techniques less frequently used in the patient with lateral patellofemoral instability. We also analyze the treatment of medial patellofemoral instability. It is a very practical book, aimed at the general orthopedic surgeon and also the ones specialized in the knee. Through a link, the surgical video techniques presented in this monograph can be accessed, with all the tips and tricks of each different author.

Contents

Chapter 1
Reconstruction of the Medial Patellofemoral Ligament: Complications After Medial Patellofemoral Ligament Reconstruction

Pieter J. Erasmus and Mathieu Thaunat

1.1 Introduction

Similar to other ligamentous reconstructions around the knee, medial patellofemoral ligament (MPFL) reconstructions can lead to complications. These complications relate to a lack of understanding of the biomechanics of the MPFL ligament and technical errors made during the reconstruction.

1.2 Biomechanics of the MPFL

The MPFL should be seen as a checkrein in preventing abnormal lateral movement of the patella, at and near full extension; it is not suppose to pull the patella medially and is of no importance once the patella has engaged the trochlea.[14]

P.J. Erasmus (✉)
University of Stellenbosch, Mediclinic,
Die Boord, Stellenbosch, South Africa
e-mail: pieter@orthoclinic.co.za

V. Sanchis-Alfonso (ed.), *Patellar Instability Surgery in Clinical Practice*, DOI 10.1007/978-1-4471-4501-1_1,
© Springer-Verlag London 2013

In the literature, on reconstruction of the MPFL, most authors suggest that the reconstructed ligament should be isometric. So-called isometric points[25,27] for the reconstruction have been suggested. However in measurements of the normal length changes in the MPFL it has repeatedly been shown to be a nonisometric ligament.[9,25,29] According to Steensen there is a 5.4 mm length change from 0° to 90° of flexion and an average of 7.2 mm length change from 0° to 120°. It is important to realize that the MPFL is a nonisometric ligament that is at its tightest at full extension and becomes more lax with flexion, as the patella engages into the trochlea.[14] Victor[33] confirmed the nonisometry of the MPFL and has suggested that there is a difference in the nonisometry of the proximal and distal fibres of the MPFL; the proximal fibres are at their tightest at full extension and the distal at 30° of flexion. In cadaveric studies it was shown that an anatomic, nonisometric, MPFL reconstruction will restore patella kinematics better than an isometric reconstruction.[22] The position of the reconstructed ligament on the patella has very little effect on the isometry of the ligament. In contrast the position on the femur has a major effect on the isometry of the ligament.[27] A more distal position increases tightness in extension and laxity in flexion; conversely a more proximal position results in a graft that is lax in extension and tight in flexion (Fig. 1.1).

In nearly all patella dislocations there are underlying causes like patella alta, trochlear dysplasia, ligamentous hyperlaxity, etc., that predisposes the patient to a patella dislocation. Patella alta seems to be the most constant predisposing factor in patella dislocations.[15] Patella height has an influence on the isometry of the MPFL, the higher the patella the bigger the nonisometry of the ligament. In unpublished cadaveric experiments we found that the average length changes in the MPFL from 0° to 90° was 4 mm. If the tibial tubercle was moved 10 mm proximally the average length change increased to 6 mm. When the tubercle was moved 10 mm distally the average length change decreased to 3 mm.[11] Considering this, it would be important to know the distance from the origin of the MPFL, at the medial epicondyle to its

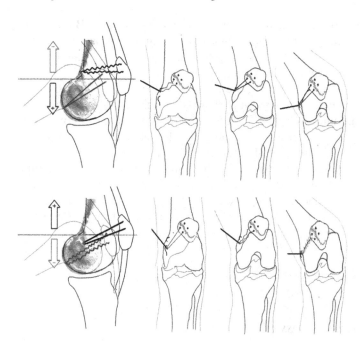

FIGURE 1.1 A proximal position on the femur will result in a graft that is loose in extension and tight in flexion. Conversely a distal femoral position will result in a graft that is tight in extension and loose in flexion

insertion on the patella, when the quads are fully contracted. The other important factor is the height of the patella in relation to the proximal sulcus. The so-called J-sign is seen[16] when near full extension the patella moves out of the trochlea and subluxes laterally. This subluxation can be caused by a short proximal trochlea or a high patella or both. At present there is no specific imaging technique to measure the length of the MPFL. The most commonly used measurements for the patella height like, Caton-Deschamps, Blackburne-Peel, and Insall-Salvati measure patella height in relation to the tibia. However, what is more important is the height of the patella in relation to the superior border of the trochlea as suggested by Bernageau and Goutallier[3] on X-rays and Biedert on MRIs.[1,4] Patella alta is associated with a long patella tendon and patella tendon length is more sensitive than Caton-Deschamps index for patella instability.[21]

In reconstructing the ligament the aim should be to use a ligament that is stronger than the original to compensate for the underlying predisposing factors which are not corrected. The reconstructed ligament should duplicate the nonisometry. The aim of the reconstruction should be to create a "favorable anisometry"[29] that duplicates that of the original ligament before injury. Failure to create favorable nonisometry can lead to redislocation, extensor lag, and loss of flexion. Loss of flexion will also lead to overload of the patella femoral joint especially of the medial facet in flexion.

1.3   Complications

1.3.1   Loss of Motion

In a long-term follow-up in our series of more than 200 MPFL reconstructions, done from 1995 till 2008, extensor lag with full passive extension and no loss of flexion was the most common complication. There was no long-term loss of flexion. Notwithstanding slight loss of active extension these patients still had an average Kujala score of 92.7 (72–100). Smith et al.[26] did a comprehensive literature research on the clinical and radiological results of MPFL reconstructions. They could only find eight papers, involving 186 MPFL reconstructions, meeting the criteria of their scoring system. In only two of these eight papers did the authors report on the postoperative range of motion and both reported on loss of flexion compared to the nonoperated leg. None reported on loss of active knee extension or extensor lag. Only one paper in this review reported on quadriceps atrophy. In this series there was an incidence of 60% quads atrophy notwithstanding a mean Kujala score of 88.6.[7] Loss of motion after an MPFL reconstruction is directly related to the tension in the reconstructed ligament. If it is too tight in extension (femoral insertion too distal) there will be an extensor lag although passive full extension will not be affected. If it is too tight in flexion (femoral insertion too proximal) there will be loss of flexion both passive and active; in this situation the patella might still be unstable in extension (Fig. 1.1).

Both the gracilis and semitendinosis tendons, generally used for reconstructing the MPFL, are stronger and stiffer than the original MPFL.[18]The strength is a positive factor considering that the underlying predisposing factors leading to the first dislocation are not corrected. The excessive stiffness however can theoretically lead to overload in the patellofemoral joint especially in cases where the reconstructed MPFL is not in the optimal position.

In our technique of MPFL reconstruction we try to recreate the normal nonisometry of the ligament, so-called favorable anisometry.[29] This creates a ligament that is tight in extension and lax in flexion. There is however the danger that the ligament can be too tight in extension resulting in an extensor lag. Postoperative quadriceps inhibition is very common and should be distinguished from a permanent extensor lag as a result of an overtight MPFL reconstruction. At 3 months postoperative follow-up there was on average a 4° (5–15°) extensor lag, probably as a result of quads inhibition, in 45% of our patients. This extensor lag was temporary and over the long term only 4 out of the more than 200 cases had permanent loss of active full extension caused by an overtight reconstruction in extension.[31]

Elias[8] has shown experimentally that a too proximally placed femoral position for the MPLF graft will lead to increased patellofemoral load with potential overload of the articular surface in the patellofemoral joint. Loss of both active and passive flexion will also be associated with this. In techniques where the aim is to have an isometric reconstructed MPFL, the danger of having a ligament that is too tight in flexion is increased. Femoral insertions near or at the adductor tubercle, although advocated by some authors, should be avoided as this will lead to a reconstruction that is too tight in flexion and too loose in extension.[23,25,27]

In prevention of motion loss complications, special attention should be given to the technique of determining the tension in the reconstructed ligament. Too much tension in the reconstructed ligament would be more detrimental, considering possible loss of motion and late patellofemoral degeneration, than too little tension. Beck showed[2] that even when applying low loads to MPFL reconstructions, it is still possible to re-establish normal translation and patellofemoral contact pressures. The aim of the MPFL reconstruction should be to restore the tension in the MPFL to the same tension that it had before being torn, with a graft that is stronger than the original ligament. If the patella of the opposite knee is stable the amount of transverse patella movement in the reconstructed patella should be similar to that of the uninjured knee. This can be achieved intraoperatively by draping both knees and comparing the amount of transverse movement. Fithian[12] advises adjusting the graft tension in such a way that a 5 lb displacing force results in 7–9 mm of lateral displacement of the patella. We recommend that the isometry of the ligament should be tested till the "favorable anisometric point" is found by using a guide pin in the proposed femoral implantation site. The "favorable anisometric point" would be a point where the reconstructed ligament will be tight in extension and lax in flexion, with a length change of about 5 mm between extension and flexion. This can be achieved, with the knee in full extension, by pulling proximally on the patella with a bone hook in the direction of the anterior superior iliac spine. In this situation the reconstructed ligament should be tight but the tension in the reconstructed ligament should be less than in the patellar tendon. This will ensure that, with maximum quads contraction, there will be more tension in the patellar tendon than in the reconstructed MPFL (Fig. 1.2). In cases of severe patella alta a distal tibial tubercle transfer should be considered as this will decrease the nonisometry of the reconstruction, allowing easier and more precise tensioning of the reconstructed ligament[11] (Fig. 1.3). We will consider a distal tubercle transfer when the Bernageau measurement is more than 8 mm or the patella tendon length is more than 60 mm, especially if this is

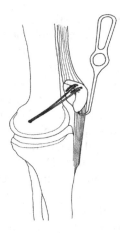

FIGURE 1.2 Tensioning the MPFL graft in full extension ensuring that the tension in the reconstruction is less than in the patellar tendon

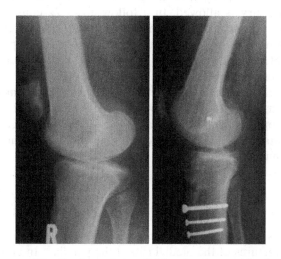

FIGURE 1.3 Distalization of the tibial tubercle combined with a MPFL reconstruction

combined with a clinically marked positive J-Sign.[16] A distal transfer of as little as 6 mm is usually adequate in these cases. Other authors have recommended different techniques for tensioning the reconstructed MPFL, the most popular being to tension the ligament between 30° and 60° of flexion when the patella is already centered in the trochlea.[5,6,20] The major length changes in the MPFL happens after 30° of flexion[25,29] and considering this, tensioning the ligament in early flexion should prevent overtensioning provided that the correct nonisometric point has been selected on the femur.

Postoperative quadriceps inhibition, although temporary, can result in an increased rehabilitation period and a late return to sporting activities. Drez[7] reported quadriceps atrophy in more than 50% of his patients at an average follow-up of 31.5 months (24–43). In an effort to combat this we start our patients on an isometric quads contraction program preoperatively. Postoperatively no braces are used and immediate active and passive full range of motion is encouraged. Isometric quadriceps exercises are continued. Full weight bearing, with the support of one or two crutches, as necessary, is allowed. In a follow-up of 22 consecutive MPFL reconstructions at an average of 29 months (8–65) we found the average side to side difference in upper leg circumference,15 cm above the knee, to be only 0.19 cm (0–1.5 cm).[11]

Should loss of motion persist for longer than 9 months after an MPFL reconstruction, we would recommend a percutaneous sequential fish scale type of tenotomy, near the implantation of the ligament on the patella, till full range of motion is restored.[31]

1.3.2   Fractures

In our series we had only three redislocations, all associated with fractures of the medial rim of the patella.[30] In all these patients the fracture occurred with a definitive injury; in two this happened in contact sport, one in soccer and the other in rugby football. The third patient sustained a redislocation when she fell off a chair trying to replace a fused light bulb. The fractures occurred respectively 2, 5, and 10 years after the initial surgery. In our reconstructing technique two 3–3.5

mm drill holes, 10 mm apart, are made on the medial edge of the patella exiting the anterior cortex approximately 6–8 mm from the medial edge. These fractures were similar to that seen in acute primary patella dislocations.[32] A gracilis autograft was used for reconstructing the ligament. This reconstructed ligament is stronger than the original MPFL and as the underlying predisposing factors have not been addressed, there will at times, be high strain on the ligament. The drill holes in the patella can act as stress raisers resulting in fractures. In all three cases the fracture involved not more than 1 cm of the medial patella. The fractures were reduced and fixed with screws all resulting in a stable patella with no longstanding sequel from the fractures.

Mikashima et al.[17] reported two fractures in 12 knees. A single transverse drill hole of 4.5 mm was made from medial to lateral through the patella. These fractures all occurred within 6 weeks from the surgery resulting in a nearly 16% incidence of fractures. Both Christiansen et al.[5] using two 4.5 mm and Gomes et al.[13] using a single 7 mm transverse drill hole reported on nontraumatic patella fractures. It is possible that too large drill holes increase the possibility of a fracture especially when they transverse the patella. Fractures of the medial rim of the patella usually do not involve the articular surface of the patella as long as they do not exit too centrally on the patella and are relatively easy to treat (Fig. 1.4). However, if this drill hole exits too far laterally it can also result in a more serious fracture (Fig. 1.5). In contrast transverse fractures, as a result of transverse drill holes will always involve the articular surface of the patella and in most cases are associated with fragmentation of the anterior cortex which makes it more serious and difficult to treat (Fig. 1.6). It can be expected that drill holes in the patella will act as stress raisers and might therefore predispose to fractures. Keeping this in mind the size and position of the drill holes should be carefully considered. Holes larger than 3.5 mm should probably be avoided. Drill holes through the medial rim should not exit too far centrally into the patella. Transverse drill holes through the patella will result in more serious fractures than drill holes through the medial rim.

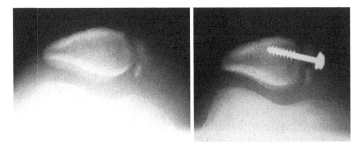

FIGURE 1.4 Redislocation after MPFL reconstruction with a fracture of the medial rim reattached with a screw and washer

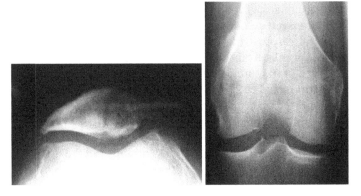

FIGURE 1.5 Central patella fracture secondary to drill hole that exit too centrally on the patella

1.3.3   Redislocations

Redislocations are rare; in the literature it varies between 0% and 4%.[5,7,24] In our series there were only three redislocations (1.5%) all associated with a fracture of the medial rim of the patella. In Smith et al.'s[26] review article there were only two post-reconstruction patella dislocations or subluxations in 186 knees; in five patients there was a positive apprehension sign.

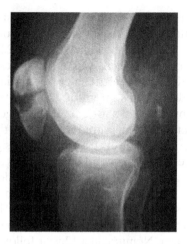

Figure 1.6 Transverse patella fracture secondary to transverse drill hole for MPFL reconstruction

1.3.4   Localized Tenderness

Localized tenderness in the region of the medial epicondyle related to either the graft or the internal fixation used, can be an irritating complication. Nomura and Inoue[19] reported an incidence of 40% as a result of using a staple for fixation just distal to the adductor tubercle. Christiansen et al.[5] reported 50% tenderness over the medial epicondyle. Steiner et al.[28] had to remove irritating screws in 10% of his patients. We[11] use a deep seated bone anchor on the medial femur and had a 6% incidence of mild localized tenderness at the exit of the graft; no surgical intervention was required.

1.3.5   Patellofemoral Degeneration

In an average 7 (4.4–9.3) year follow-up of our first 29 patients[10] the Tegner (5.8), Lysholm (88.5), and IKDC (81) scores were statistically unchanged at 3, 5, and 7 years follow-up. Patellofemoral cartilage damage at the time of the

MPFL reconstruction had a negative effect on the Lysholm score but no effect on the Tegner and IKDC scores. In a separate 29 (8–54) month follow-up study of 22 consecutive MPFL reconstructions[9] there was no statistical correlation between the Kujala score, trochlea dysplasia, and Caton Deschamps index. In this group of 22 patients there was a weak correlation between a lower score; a longer patella tendon and a higher patella, measured according to the Bernageau technique. There was however a statistically significant correlation between patellofemoral degeneration at the time of the reconstruction and a low Kujala score. It does seem that development of patellofemoral degeneration can be prevented by an isolated MPFL reconstruction. The effect on patellofemoral degeneration present at the time of the reconstruction is unclear. Nomura, in a 12 year follow-up, reported similar results.[20]

1.4   Summary

Medial patellofemoral ligament (MPFL) reconstructions have good results with few complications notwithstanding varied techniques used. Biomechanical and technical principles should be adhered to in preventing complications. The reconstructed MPFL should be tight in extension and lax in flexion. In cases of severe patella alta, a distalization of the tibial tubercle should be considered. With maximum quadriceps contraction the tension in the patellar tendon should be more than the tension in the reconstructed ligament. Drill holes in the patella should be through the medial rim preferably not exceeding 3.5 mm in diameter. Prominence of the reconstructed graft or fixation material over the medial condyle will lead to localized tenderness and is easily avoided by using nonprominent fixation devices. There seems to be no progression in patellofemoral degeneration after MPFL reconstructions, in follow-up periods of 7–12 years.

References

1. Barnett A, Prentice M, Mandalia V. The patellotrochlear index: a more clinically relevant measurement of patella height? J Bone Joint Surg. 2009;91-B:413.
2. Beck P, Brown NA, Greis PE, et al. Patellofemoral contact pressures and lateral patellar translation after medial patellofemoral ligament reconstruction. Am J Sports Med. 2007;35:1557-63.
3. Bernageau J, Goutallier D. Exam radiologique de l'articulation femorale-patellaire.L'actualite rhumatologique. Paris: Expansion Scientifique Francaise; 1984.
4. Biedert R, Albrecht S. The patellotrochlear index: a new index for assessing patellar height. Knee Surg Sports Traumatol Arthrosc. 2006;14:707-12.
5. Christiansen SE, Jacobsen BW, Lund B, et al. Reconstruction of the medial patellofemoral ligament with gracilis tendon autograft in transverse patellar drill holes. Arthroscopy. 2008;24:82-7.
6. Deie M, Ochi Y, Sumen M, et al. Reconstruction of the medial patellofemoral ligament for the treatment of habitual or recurrent dislocation of the patella in children. J Bone Joint Surg. 2003;85:887-90.
7. Drez D, Edwards TB, Williams CS. Results of medial patellofemoral ligament reconstruction in the treatment of patella dislocation. Arthroscopy. 2001;17:298-306.
8. Elias JJ, Cosgarea AJ. Technical errors during MPFL reconstruction could overload the medial patello femoral cartilage. Am J Sports Med. 2006;34:1478-85.
9. Erasmus PJ (1998) Reconstruction of the medial patellofemoral ligament in recurrent dislocation of the patella. ISAKOS Buenos Aires May 1997 [abstract]. Arthroscopy. 1998;14(Suppl):S42.
10. Erasmus PJ. Long term follow-up of MPFL reconstruction. Washington: American Orthopedic Society for Sport Medicine (AOSS); 2005.
11. Erasmus PJ. Influence of patella height on the results of MPFL reconstruction. Florence: ISAKOS; 2007.
12. Fithian DC, Gupta N. Patellar instability: principles of soft tissue repair and reconstruction. Tech Knee Surg. 2006;5:19-26.
13. Gomes EJ, Marczyk LS, de Cesar PC, et al. Medial patellofemoral ligament reconstruction with semitendinosus autograft for chronic patellar instability: follow-up study. Arthroscopy. 2004;20: 147-51.

14. Heegaard J, Leyvraz PF, Van Kampen A, et al. Influence of soft tissue structure on patella three dimensional tracking. Clin Orthop Relat Res. 1996;299:235-43.
15. Hvid I, Andersen L, Schmidt H. Patellar height and femoral trochlea development. Acta Orthop Scand. 1983;54:91-3.
16. Johnson JJ, van Dyk EG, Green JR, et al. Clinical assessment of asymptomatic knees: comparison of men and women. Arthroscopy. 1998;22:787-93.
17. Mikashima Y, Kimura M, Komayashi Y, et al. Clinical results of isolated reconstruction of the medial patellofemoral ligament for recurrent dislocation and subluxation of the patella. Acta Orthop Belg. 2006;72:65-71.
18. Mountney J, Senavongse W, Amis AA, et al. Tensile strength of the medial patellofemoral ligament before and after repair or reconstruction. J Bone Joint Surg. 2005;87:36-40.
19. Nomura E, Inoue M. Hybrid medial patellofemoral ligament reconstruction using semitendinosis tendon for recurrent patellar dislocation: minimum 3 years follow up. Arthroscopy. 2006;22:787-93.
20. Nomura E, Motoyasu I, Kobayashi S. Long-term follow-up and knee osteoarthritis change after medial patellofemoral ligament reconstruction for recurrent patellar dislocation. Am J Sports Med. 2007;35:1851-8.
21. Neyret P, Robinson AH, Le Coultre B, et al. Patella tendon length – the factor in patella instability? Knee. 2002;9:3-6.
22. Parker DA, Alexander JW, Conditt MA, et al. Comparison of isometric and anatomic reconstruction of the medial patellofemoral ligament: a cadaveric study. Orthopedics. 2008;31:339-43.
23. Sillanpää PJ, Mäempää H, Matilla W, et al. A mini-invasive adductor magnus tendon transfer technique for medial patellofemoral ligament reconstruction: a technical note. Knee Surg Sports Traumatol Arthrosc. 2009;17:508-12.
24. Schöttle PB, Fucentese SF, Romero J. Clinical and radiological outcome of medial patellofemoral ligament reconstruction with a semitendinosis autograft for patella instability. Knee Surg Sports Traumatol Arthrosc. 2005;13:516-21.
25. Smirk C, Morris H. The anatomy and reconstruction of the medial patellofemoral ligament. Knee. 2003;10:221-7.
26. Smith TO, Walker J, Russel N. Outcomes of medial patellofemoral ligament reconstruction for patellar instability: a systemic review. Knee Surg Sports Traumatol Arthrosc. 2007;15:1301-14.
27. Steensen RN, Dopirak RM, McDonald WG. The anatomy and isometry of the medial patello femoral joint. Am J Sports Med. 2004;32:1509-13.
28. Steiner TM, Torga-Spak R, Teitge RA. Medial patellofemoral ligament reconstruction in patients with lateral patella instability and trochlear dysplasia. Am J Sports Med. 2006;34:1254-61.

29. Thaunat M, Erasmus PJ. The favourable anisometry: an original concept for medial patellofemoral ligament reconstruction. Knee. 2007;9:3-6.
30. Thaunat M, Erasmus PJ. Recurrent patella dislocation after medial patellofemoral reconstruction. Knee Surg Sports Traumatol Arthrosc. 2008;16:40-3.
31. Thaunat M, Erasmus PJ. Management of overtight medial patell-ofemoral ligament reconstruction. Knee Surg Sports Traumatol Arthrosc. 2009;17:480-3.
32. Toritsuka Y, Horibe S, Hiro-Oka A, et al. Medial marginal fracture of the patella following patellar dislocation. Knee. 2007;14:429-33.
33. Victor J, Wong P, Witvrouw E, et al. How isometric are the medial patellofemoral, superficial medial collateral, and lateral collateral ligaments of the knee? Am J Sports Med. 2009;37:2028-36.

Chapter 2
Reconstruction of the Medial Patellofemoral Ligament: How I Do It

Eric W. Edmonds and Donald C. Fithian

2.1 Introduction

Reconstruction of the medial patellofemoral ligament (MPFL) has been described utilizing a myriad of fixation techniques. We have elected to utilize a technique that secures the graft to the femur with an interference screw and secures the graft to the patella by suturing it to itself after threading it through bone tunnels. This allows for easy tensioning of the graft while not sacrificing fixation.

2.2 Indications

Recurrent episodic patellofemoral instability is the primary indication for MPFL reconstruction. It is indicated for patients with at least two documented patellar dislocations and a physical examination demonstrating excessive lateral patellar motion. Examination must demonstrate excessive

E.W. Edmonds (✉)
Department of Orthopaedic Surgery, University of California,
San Diego, CA, USA

Pediatric Orthopaedic and Scoliosis Center,
Rady Children's Hospital San Diego,
San Diego, CA, USA
e-mail: ericwedmonds@yahoo.com

V. Sanchis-Alfonso (ed.), *Patellar Instability Surgery in Clinical Practice*, DOI 10.1007/978-1-4471-4501-1_2,
© Springer-Verlag London 2013

laxity of the medial retinacular ligaments and is evaluated by applying lateral and medial forces (about 5 lb) to the patella with the knee in 30° of flexion. In this position of flexion, in normal knees, the patella sits close to the center of the femoral groove. Increased laxity is signified by >2 quadrants of translation, or >10 mm lateral translation from the resting position. Examination under anesthesia may be necessary to accomplish this task.

2.3   Contraindications

Randomized studies have shown no significant benefit of surgery for first-time patellar dislocation, unless there is a loose body secondary to patella instability.[1,2] Furthermore, trochlear dysplasia (prominent or flat trochlea) may call for additional procedures to reduce joint forces, offload cartilage defects, and/or enhance patellar stability. A complete examination should evaluate the patient for associated injuries and rule out other potential causes of sudden knee pain and giving way. ACL injuries, meniscal tears, cartilage flap tears and defects, degenerative joint disease, and plica are just a few pathologies that have been mistaken for patellar instability.

2.4   Surgical Technique Step by Step

2.4.1   Positioning and EUA

The patient is positioned supine on a standard table. A sterile bump can be placed under the knee to keep the knee slightly flexed. If a diagnostic arthroscopy is performed before MPFL reconstruction, then the limb is placed in a low profile adjustable leg holder to adjust knee flexion during the procedure. Exam under anesthesia should always be performed during positioning to confirm excessive lateral patellar mobility. This is defined as an absent checkrein sign, >2 quadrants lateral excursion, or >10 mm lateral excursion at 30° of flexion.

It is often advantageous to use image intensifier to confirm the femoral attachment sight of the MPFL radiographically and therefore patient positioning should consider convenient placement of the image intensifier.

2.4.2   Diagnostic Arthroscopy

Arthroscopy is used to address articular lesions and stage degenerative changes. Standard anterolateral and anteromedial portals are used. If necessary, a superolateral portal is used to facilitate additional viewing of the patellar articular surface and passive patellar tracking and mobility. At this time, the patellofemoral compartment is assessed for the severity of articular cartilage injury and the presence of degenerative changes. Unstable cartilage flaps are debrided and loose bodies addressed.

2.4.3   Graft Harvest

Having confirmed that the medial retinacular structures are incompetent by examination, the next step following arthroscopy is harvesting the semitendinosis autograft. Utilizing bony landmarks, the pes anserine is identified and a longitudinal incision is made in the skin of approximately 2.5 cm using a #15 blade scalpel (Fig. 2.1). Dissection is carried down to the sartorius fascia and a blunt finger sweep is performed to expose the fascia and help identify the location of the underlying gracilis and semitendinosis tendons. An incision in line with the semitendinosis is then made through the sartorius fascia to gain access to the semitendinosis tendon. Only the semitendinosis is harvested as the graft should be 240 mm to make a 120 mm-doubled graft and the gracilis is often of insufficient length.

The semitendinosis is harvested using a closed tendon stripper after detaching the distal end from the tibia, securing the graft using 0 vicryl suture, and freeing the tendon from its

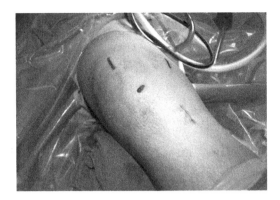

FIGURE 2.1 Intraoperative photograph demonstrating standard incisions for MPFL reconstruction, including: two anterior para-patellar arthroscopy portals, tibial incision for hamstring autograft harvest, medial patella incision, and medial distal femur incision

fascial attachment to the medial gastrocnemius. The graft is taken to the back-table and debrided of remaining muscular tissue. The proximal end is then secured and tubularized in a similar fashion to the distal end. The graft is then doubled over and that end is whip-stitched for 20–25 mm with 0 vicryl to tubularize the graft, which is then left on the back table in a saline-soaked sponge.

2.4.4   Patella Exposure

A 2.5 cm incision is then made over the medial one third of the patella. The deep bursal layer is incised to expose the longitudinal fibers (layer 1) of the extensor retinaculum. The medial third of the patella, from the medial border of the patellar tendon to the insertion of the MPFL, is exposed subperiosteally. This dissection is best carried out with a sharp #15 scalpel. Care should be taken to remain subperiosteal as you turn the corner at the medial border of the patella. Continue the dissection through the MPFL fibers (layer 2), which can be identified as they course horizontally into the proximal medial two thirds of the patella. The dissection should remain extra-articular. The layer deep to the MPFL is layer 3, which is the joint capsule. After the MPFL is released, blunt dissection with a long clamp is used to develop a plane medially between the MPFL and the capsular layer.

These horizontal fibers of the MPFL are about 1-cm wide and run at a right angle to the longitudinal fibers of layer 1. This is an extra-articular plane between the medial retinaculum superficially and the joint capsule on the deep surface. The vastus medialis obliquus (VMO) tendon lies superficially. The tunnel for the MPFL graft will be placed at this level.

The plane of soft tissue dissection through the retinaculum is important. The key is to avoid dissecting too deeply into the joint, because passing the graft through the joint space is nonanatomic, can interfere with healing, and may cause joint abrasion or mechanical abrasion to the graft as it passes over the medial femur during motion and activity. It is best to dissect between layers 2 and 3. This is an easy plane to develop and allows reapproximation of the native MPFL over the graft during closure. Also acceptable is a tunnel superficial to the MPFL, between layers 1 and 2. However, the superficial surface of the MPFL is adherent to the overlying VMO insertion and layer 1, so this plane is more difficult to develop than the deeper interval.

2.4.5   Patella Bone Tunnels

After approaching the patella, bone tunnels in the anterior medial patella are created. Using a 3.2 or 4.5 mm drill bit, depending on graft thickness, two bone tunnels are made in the proximal half of the patella. Start by creating two anterior holes placed 5–7 mm from the medial edge of the patella. These holes are drilled approximately 10 mm in depth. Next, two medial holes aiming laterally should connect with holes just created on the anterior surface of the patella (on a right knee, these should correspond with 1 and 3 o'clock). The starting point on the medial edge of the patella for these holes corresponds with the insertion point of the MPFL, again deep to layer 2, deep to the VMO, but superficial to the joint capsule. A small angled curette is used to complete this connection and create the tunnel.

2.4.6   Femur Exposure

After the patella bone tunnels are prepared, a second incision 3 cm long is made centered over the medial epicondyle to approach the femoral MPFL origin. After incising the skin and subcutaneous tissue the medial epicondyle is easily palpated and blunt dissection with digital palpation confirms the relative location. The native MPFL originates on the ridge between the adductor tubercle and the medial femoral epicondyle at a point 9 mm proximal and 5 mm posterior to the medial epicondyle. The Bieth pin for the femoral tunnel will be placed at this point.

2.4.7   Femoral Tunnel

Placement of the femoral attachment is one of the most critical steps of the operation. The isometry and behavior of the MPFL is far more affected by the femoral insertion site than the patella site. Radiographically, the pin is placed at the junction of Blumensat's line and posterior femoral cortex. If placed at this described clinical and radiographic position, then the isometry of the MPFL should be close to physiologic (as this corresponds to its femoral origin in anatomic dissection). Fine tuning may be required and isometry should be verified by passing a suture through the tissue tunnel created with a clamp between the patellar and femoral incisions. (This same suture will be used as a shuttle to take the graft through the tissue tunnel later). The suture is looped over the femoral Bieth pin and through the patella bone tunnels (Fig. 2.2). The knee is then put through a full range of motion while holding the suture with a hemostat. If the suture tightens as you flex the knee, then keep the first Bieth pin in place and place a second pin slightly distal on the femur. If the

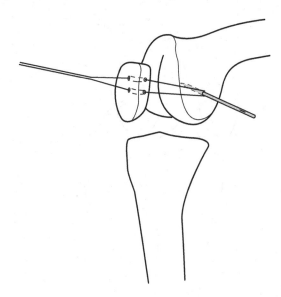

FIGURE 2.2 Line drawing demonstrating assessment of isometric point on femur utilizing Bieth pin and suture passed through patella tunnels

suture tightens as you extend the knee, then keep the first Bieth pin in place and place a second pin more proximal on the femur. Recheck isometry to ensure the patella tracks smoothly in the trochlear without excess constraint throughout its range.[3-5]

With the isometric point confirmed, the femoral tunnel can now be drilled over the Bieth pin to a depth of 25 mm with the appropriate diameter reamer, dependent on the thickness of the doubled part of the graft (usually about 6–7 mm).

2.4.8   Graft Placement

Pass the doubled end of graft into the femoral tunnel by pulling the Bieth pin medially and secure it in place with an appropriately sized interference screw (Fig. 2.3). Ensure that

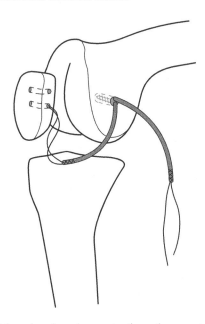

Figure 2.3 Line drawing demonstrating placement of graft into femoral tunnel, secured using interference screw

the graft does not twist to avoid knotting the tissue on the medial femur. Pass the two free ends of the graft through the soft tissue tunnel created earlier using the shuttle suture (Fig. 2.4). Each limb is passed through a patella bone tunnel, folded over and sewn to itself with nonabsorbable suture (Fig. 2.5). This patella two bone tunnel technique allows for titration of patellar constraint fixing the graft at the perfect length that allows no excess slack and no excess tension. Tensioning the graft is one of the most important steps in the procedure and care should be taken to avoid overtensioning the graft while obtaining adequate fixation. The length should be set such that a firm endpoint is felt as the patella is translated laterally preventing dislocation. This is done by confirming normal translation laterally (<10 mm or 2 quadrants) with a firm end point at 30° knee flexion. No tension should be felt before the end point is reached. The patella

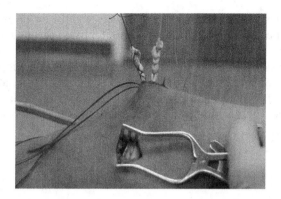

FIGURE 2.4 Intraoperative photograph demonstrating graft in place after passage between two working incisions ready for placement through patellar tunnels and tensioning

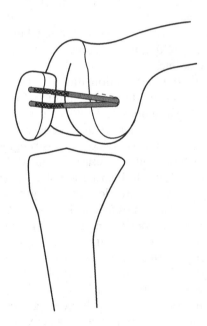

FIGURE 2.5 Line drawing demonstrating secured graft, sutured onto itself, post-tensioning, at the completion of the MPFL reconstruction

should smoothly engage the trochlea slightly on its lateral side in early flexion and track without tension throughout its range.

Incision closure is then started by first utilizing Vicryl to repair layers #2 and #1 over the top of the graft and patella. Then, absorbable skin sutures are used to perform a layered closure of the three incisions and the two arthroscopy portals.

2.5   Postoperative Management

Outpatient management is the norm for this procedure. A femoral nerve block placed intraoperatively and oral narcotics are used for pain control. A knee range of motion brace is used for 4–6 weeks to prevent falls. Immediate full weight bearing is allowed and gait may be progressed as soon as good muscular control has been established. Physical therapy is needed to restore quadriceps control and range of motion as quickly as possible.

The principles of rehabilitation after MPFL reconstruction are similar to those guiding rehabilitation following other ligamentous reconstructions of the knee, such as anterior cruciate ligament (ACL). The keys are to address pain control, range of motion (ROM), quadriceps strengthening, and proximal lower limb control. Return of full ROM, pain control, and protected weight-bearing are stressed in the early phases of recovery. Progression of strength training and return to functional activities follows lines of evidence regarding graft necrosis, remodeling, and tunnel ingrowth which are most commonly associated with ACL reconstruction. We emphasize early, controlled ROM to reduce pain, prevent scar formation and capsular contractions, and to re-establish full ROM (particularly extension). Proximal control is enhanced by performing nonweight-bearing exercises targeting the hip abductors, external rotators, and extensors. Patients are encouraged to return to their sport or activity once they can achieve satisfactory single limb dynamic control.

2.6   Pearls and Pitfalls

A pitfall to this procedure is patient selection. Remember that sudden anterior knee pain with instability is a nonspecific complaint and that this procedure should be done only to reconstruct laxity of the medial retinaculum and MPFL. Examination under anesthesia may be necessary to confirm this laxity.

A pitfall during surgery is a short graft. Inadequate graft length will not allow for proper constraint to be applied to the patella and can lead to overtensioning of the graft and subsequent failure or pain. In these rare cases, when the semitendinosis is too short, the gracilis can be harvested, as well. They are then sewn together at their insertional stumps and the joined end is fashioned as if it were the looped end of a doubled semitendinosis graft. Furthermore, an allograft semitendinosis can be used and should be prepared in the same fashion as the autograft. The pearl for allograft choice is to select a graft of sufficient length, as described.

A pitfall of tunnel placement is to make the bone bridge between the holes too narrow and fracturing the bone tunnels may occur. A pearl, if a fracture occurs, is to then place a more lateral bone tunnel. Alternatively, the graft can be fixed in the patella with an interference screw and careful graft tension applied through a transpatellar suture shuttled laterally on a Bieth pin, or secured using suture anchors if adequate fixation exists in the remaining patella.

A pearl to tunnel placement of the femoral tunnel is that this step is the most critical step of the procedure. The isometric behavior of the MPFL is far more affected by the femoral insertion site than the patella site. The native MPFL sees greatest tension in full knee extension with the quadriceps contracted. The ideal length change behavior, or isometry, for an MPFL graft has not been established. It is probably not necessary that the graft be perfectly isometric, but checking isometry will help the surgeon understand how the graft is behaving during knee motion and also verify that no untoward effect is seen. It is important to ensure that the graft is not overtightened. The graft should have no tension and no slack, acting as a passive constraint just as it does in normal physiology. An objective firm endpoint should be felt as the patella is translated about 7 mm laterally, but no tension should be felt before that point when the knee is flexed 30°.

Excessive tension will lead to early failure, pain, and medial patellar degenerative changes. Excessive laxity will not restore stability to the patella. We fix the graft to the patella with the knee at 30° flexion, with the patella centered passively in the trochlea. Care is taken to remove all slack from the graft, but the graft should be under no tension whatsoever when the patella is centered in the groove.

2.7   Complications

As mentioned in the section on "Pitfalls," fracturing of the patella may occur; however, in contrast to procedures that place an interference screw and require full width drilling of the patella, this technique weakens only the medial proximal quadrant of the patella and risk of fracturing is likely less. Besides this specific complication, the standard risks of operative intervention exist such as infection, blood loss, neurologic injury, and anesthetic complications, but all are very minimal risks.

Postoperatively, one of the biggest potential complications is knee stiffness. If the patient has not regained at least 0–90° of knee flexion by postoperative week 6, then the recommendation is to increase the intensity of the physical therapy program. Manipulation under anesthesia to regain that motion by week 9 may be done if the stiffness is not resolved by that time.

References

1. Andrade A, Thomas N. Randomized comparison of operative vs. nonoperative treatment following first time dislocation. European Society for Sports, Knee and Arthroscopy, Rome. 2002.

2. Nikku R, Nietosvaara Y, Kallio PE, et al. Operative versus closed treatment of primary dislocation of the patella: similar 2-year results in 125 randomized patients. Acta Orthop Scand. 1997;68:419-23.
3. Nomura E, Inoue M, Osada N. Anatomical analysis of the medial patellofemoral ligament of the knee, especially at the femoral attachment. Knee Surg Sports Traumatol Arthrosc. 2005;13:510-5.
4. Schöttle PB, Schmeling A, Rosenstiel N, et al. Radiographic landmarks for femoral tunnel placement in medial patellofemoral ligament reconstruction. Am J Sports Med. 2007;35:801-4.
5. Steensen RN, Dopirak RM, McDonald WG 3rd. The anatomy and isometry of the medial patellofemoral ligament: implications for reconstruction. Am J Sports Med. 2004;32:1509-13.

Chapter 3
Reconstruction of the Medial Patellofemoral Ligament: How I Do It

Robert A. Teitge and Roger Torga-Spak

3.1 Introduction

The medial patellofemoral ligament (MPFL) has been recognized as the primary stabilizer against lateral patellar dislocation or subluxation.[2,4,5] Consequently if there is lateral patellar instability there is also an insufficient MPFL. Various reconstruction procedures of the MPFL using adductor magnus,[1,10] quadriceps tendon,[8] semitendinosus,[5] gracilis,[2,3] and synthetic tissue[6] have been recently developed.

The technique we postulate follows the same basic principles of all ligament reconstruction: (1) selection of a sufficiently strong and stiff graft, (2) isometric graft placement, (3) correct tension, (4) adequate fixation, and (5) no condylar rubbing or impingement. Adductor longus tendon was used in most of our reconstructions, whereas quadriceps tendon autograft or bone patellar tendon allograft was preferred in cases with trochlear dysplasia based on the concept that a

R. Torga-Spak (✉)
Faculty of Orthopaedics and Traumatology,
Department of Surgery, Instituto Universitario CEMIC,
Buenos Aires, Argentina
e-mail: rtorgaspak@gmail.com

V. Sanchis-Alfonso (ed.), *Patellar Instability Surgery in Clinical Practice,* DOI 10.1007/978-1-4471-4501-1_3,
© Springer-Verlag London 2013

stronger structure is needed to compensate for inadequate support provided by a flat trochlea.

3.2   Indications

Reconstruction of the MPFL is a very common procedure in our practice for the treatment of lateral patellar instability. We indicate the isolated reconstruction of the MPFL as the procedure of choice for three different clinical pictures: (1) when no underlying alignment or morphologic abnormality is identified; (2) when many underlying subtle alignment or morphologic abnormalities are identified (i.e., increased femoral anteversion, patella alta, trochlear dysplasia, and genu valgum), but it is not possible to detect which of these deformities contribute the most to the instability; and (3) when one underlying alignment or morphologic abnormality is identified (i.e., increased femoral anteversion or trochlear dysplasia), but the magnitude and the risks of the procedure to correct that deformity outweigh its potential benefits.

3.3   Surgical Technique

3.3.1   Graft Selection and Harvesting

The adductor magnus with its insertion just proximal to the medial epicondyle can be conveniently used to reconstruct the MPFL. With the knee in extension a 4- to 6-cm skin incision is performed midway between the medial epicondyle and medial edge of the patella. Dissection is carried through the subcutaneous fat and fascia over the vastus medialis is opened. The vastus medialis is elevated off the intermuscular septum, which is then split longitudinally to expose the adductor tendon (Fig. 3.1). A tendon stripper is used to strip the adductor magnus tendon and a whipstitch (approximately 10 cm long) is placed in the free end. The diameter is then measured by passing it through a sizer, most conveniently a 3.5 or 4.5 drill sleeve.

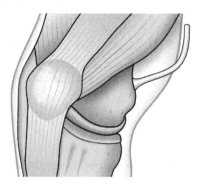

FIGURE 3.1 Harvesting of the adductor magnus tendon

3.3.2 Isometric Location

The graft must be located isometrically to avoid overstretching it to failure during joint motion or overconstraining patellar motion. A transverse 2.5-mm hole is placed through the patella far anteriorly at about the junction of the proximal and mid one-third height. A 1.5-cm incision is made on the lateral side of the patella and a strand of #2 Vicryl is passed through the hole with a small loop tied on the medial aspect to pass over a 2.5-mm Kirschner wire, which is inserted into bone near the medial epicondyle. A pneumatic Isometer (Synthes, Paoli, Pa) is inserted into the hole in the lateral patella and the #2 Vicryl isometric measurement suture is passed through. The knee is placed through a full range of motion while the change in length between the medial epicondylar K-wire and the medial border of the patella is read on the isometer (Fig. 3.2). The string tension is set at 3 lb. Adjustments in the position of the K-wire around the medial epicondyle are made until no excursion is read on the isometer during the full range of knee motion. Once the isometric point is located, a tunnel is drilled from the insertion of the adductor tendon to the isometric measurement point and the graft is pulled through this tunnel. A second tunnel the diameter of the graft is drilled through the patella at the site of the

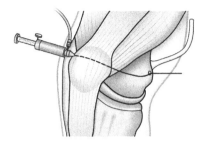

FIGURE 3.2 Location of the isometric point on the medial epicondyle

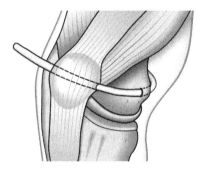

FIGURE 3.3 Graft passing through the tunnel in the medial epicon-dyle and through the patellar tunnel

2.5-mm hole used to measure isometry. The graft is passed deep to the vastus medialis, exiting the tunnel in the medial condyle anteriorly, and then pulled into the patellar tunnel (Fig. 3.3).

3.3.3   Correct Tension

The ligament is not a dynamic structure that pulls the patella medially, but rather a static restraint that prevents is from moving too far laterally. The tension set in the graft must be

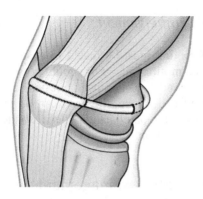

FIGURE 3.4 Graft sutured to the quadriceps expansion on the anterior aspect of the patella

enough to limit lateral excursion to an amount that approximates that of the normal contralateral knee. Tension is set with the knee flexed 60–90° to hold the patella centered in the trochlea and to avoid risk of pulling it too far medial. Tension should not be set with the knee in extension and the patella outside the trochlea, as no reference exists to determine where it is centered.

3.3.4   Secure Fixation

Tendon through bone tunnel provides the greatest stable fixation, and an adequate bone tunnel can be placed transversely through the patella with 3.5-, 4.5- or 6-mm drills depending on the diameter of the graft. After passing the graft from medial to lateral it is turned superficially onto the anterior surface of the patella where it is sutured to the medial retinaculum where it enters the patella, the lateral retinaculum where it exits, and the quadriceps expansion. If the graft is long enough, extra sutures can be placed from its free end to the medial tendon before it enters the patellar tunnel (Fig. 3.4).

3.3.5   Avoid Impingement

The range of motion must be tested to ensure unrestricted patellar or knee motion. The graft should not rub against the medial femoral condyle. If impingement on the medial femoral condyle wall is detected, the graft can be placed on the anterior surface of the patella and pulled into the lateral tunnel in a medial direction.

3.4   Postoperative Management

Postoperative treatment includes full range of motion, full weight bearing, continuous passive motion, and active exercises, with avoidance of stairs, squatting, and resistive leg extension until the tendon has healed into the tunnel. A knee brace in extension is used for ambulation during the first 3–6 weeks to protect against falling due to quadriceps inhibition

3.5   Our Experience

Reconstruction of the MPFL has been performed in our institution since 1982 in more than 300 patients. We have recently evaluated the clinical results of MPFL reconstruction in 34 patients with chronic patellar instability and trochlear dysplasia.[9] Patients were followed for a mean 66.5 months. There were 85.3% and 91.1% good and excellent results based on Kujala and Lysholm scores, respectively. No recurrent dislocations have occurred.

3.6   Complications

Patellar fracture at the transverse stress riser has occurred in the early postoperative period as a result of falling onto the flexed knee in a couple of patients. Another patient had graft advancement after loosening in a high-speed motor vehicle accident 5 months after reconstruction. Although we check isometry routinely, in a few patients the graft was found to be too tight in flexion in the early postoperative period. These patients complained of tension and pain in the medial aspect of the knee and improved immediately after arthroscopic release of the graft.

References

1. Avikainen VJ, Nikku RK, Seppanen-Lehmonen TK. Adductor magnus tenodesis for patellar dislocation. Technique and preliminary results. Clin Orthop Relat Res. 1993;297:12-6.
2. Conlan T, Garth WP Jr, Lemons JE. Evaluation of the medial soft-tissue restraints of the extensor mechanism of the knee. J Bone Joint Surg Am. 1993;75:682-93.
3. Christiansen SE, Jacobsen BW, Lund B, et al. Reconstruction of the medial patellofemoral ligament with gracilis tendon autograft in transverse patellar drill holes. Arthroscopy. 2008;24:82-7.
4. Desio SM, Burks RT, Bachus KN. Soft tissue restraints to lateral patellar translation in the human knee. Am J Sports Med. 1998;26:59-65.
5. Hautamaa PV, Fithian DC, Kaufman KR, et al. Medial soft tissue restraints in lateral patellar instability and repair. Clin Orthop Relat Res. 1998;349:174-82.
6. Nomura E, Inoue M. Hybrid medial patellofemoral ligament reconstruction using the semitendinous tendon for recurrent patellar dislocation: minimum 3 years' follow-up. Arthroscopy. 2006;22:787-93.
7. Nomura E, Horiuchi Y, Kihara M. A mid-term follow-up of medial patellofemoral ligament reconstruction using an artificial ligament for recurrent patellar dislocation. Knee. 2000;7:211-5.
8. Steensen RN, Dopirak RM, Maurus PB. A simple technique for reconstruction of the medial patellofemoral ligament using a quadriceps tendon graft. Arthroscopy. 2005;21:365-70.
9. Steiner TM, Torga-Spak R, Teitge RA. Medial patellofemoral ligament reconstruction in patients with lateral patellar instability and trochlear dysplasia. Am J Sports Med. 2006;34:1254-61.
10. Teitge R, Torga-Spak R. Medial patellofemoral ligament reconstruction. Orthopedics. 2004;27:1037-40.

Chapter 4
Combined Tibial Tubercle Realignment and MPFL Reconstruction

Joan C. Monllau, Xavier Pelfort, Pablo Gelber, and Marc Tey

4.1 Introduction

The etiology of the patellar instability involves multiple factors and it can often be successfully managed with conservative treatment. This is particularly so in cases of primary dislocation. If there is no clinical improvement with nonoperative management, surgery may be considered especially in cases of recurrent patellar dislocation. In these patients, a complete physical examination and some imaging studies are mandatory. With regards physical examination, some risk factors such as Q angle increase, *vastus medialis obliquus* insufficiency, joint laxity, previous surgery, malalignment, or torsion deformities are special concerns that need to be ruled out.[11]

J.C. Monllau (✉)
Department of Orthopaedic Surgery and Traumatology,
Hospital de la Santa Creu i Sant Pau,
Universitat Autònoma de Barcelona,
Barcelona, Spain

Arthroscopy Unit, ICATME, Institut Universitari Dexeus,
Universitat Autònoma de Barcelona,
Barcelona, Spain
e-mail: jmonllau@santpau.cat

V. Sanchis-Alfonso (ed.), *Patellar Instability Surgery in Clinical Practice,* DOI 10.1007/978-1-4471-4501-1_4,
© Springer-Verlag London 2013

The medial patellofemoral ligament (MPFL) is an extracapsular fascial band that lies within the second of three layers on the medial side of the knee. It has been shown that after a patellar dislocation, a tear to the MPFL occurs in 94% of the patients.[12] For this reason, meticulous assessment of the MPFL is crucial. With the knee at 20–30° of flexion, the examiner tries to subluxate the patella laterally. MPFL deficiency is suspected if the patient is apprehensive during this maneuvre. Furthermore, a specific imaging protocol which includes: conventional radiographs to evaluate patellar height, morphology and osteochondral fractures of the patella, computed tomography scan to assess patellar tilt, TT-TG measurement, and femoral as well as tibial torsion must be done. Magnetic resonance images, to particularly evaluate the MPFL and patellar chondral injuries, should also be performed in all cases of patellar instability.

4.2   Indications and Contraindications

Due to the broad spectrum of etiologies and allied conditions, the surgical treatment of patellar instability should be individualized. Patients with a history of recurrent patellar dislocation, disruption of the MPFL on the MRI, a positive test for MPFL insufficiency on physical examination, and an increased TT-TG distance more than 20 mm are the optimal indications for performing a distal realignment combined with a MPFL reconstruction. As do some others,[13] the authors do not consider trochlear dysplasia, lateral femoral condyle dysplasia, or *patella alta* as contraindications for this procedure.

4.3   Surgical Technique

The patient is placed in the supine position on the operating table. A high lateral post is used to stabilize the lower extremity. The injured knee is flexed approximately at 90° and maintained with a foot bump. A well-padded tourniquet tied on the proximal operative thigh is recommended.

4.3.1   Distal Tibial Tubercle Realignment

An anterior longitudinal incision is made from the distal part of the patellar tendon and extending distally around 10 cm following the anterior ridge of the tibia. The patellar tendon is identified and then a subcutaneous lateral patellar retinacular release is performed. Afterward, the patellar tendon tibial attachment as well as the tibial tuberosity (TT) is exposed. For an adequate TT osteotomy, a distal dissection of from 6 to 7 cm is prepared. Two Kirschner wires are drilled to guide the bone cut at the upper and lower part of the TT. Similarly to the osteotomy described by Fulkerson,[2,3] the superior wire is drilled in a 45° oblique direction, with reference to the antero-posterior axis of the tibia, aiming toward the posterolateral tibial corner. This obliquity in the proximal part of the osteotomy is responsible for the anteriorization of the TT at the time it slides medially. On the distal half of the osteotomy, the second wire is drilled in a more perpendicular direction (70° to 80° with respect to anteroposterior axis of the tibia). In this way, the bone cut will get thinner downward as it goes distally. Consequently, the distal part of the osteotomized TT will be more medially than anteriorly moved. Excessive anterior prominence of the TT at the distal part after surgery should be avoided. Subsequently, two 4.5 mm holes are predrilled on the anterior cortex of the TT for later lag-screw compression fixation of the osteotomized bone. Afterward, the TT osteotomy is performed with the help of an oscillating saw and osteotomes. This is when the patellar height can be modified if needed by moving and fixing the osteotomized TT either more distally or proximally on the sagittal plane. After placing the TT in the desired final position, fixation is performed by drilling the second tibial cortex with a 3.5 mm drill and using two cortical 4.5 mm lag compression screws. Once distal realignment is completed, MPFL reconstruction can proceed.

4.3.2   MPFL Reconstruction

MPFL reconstruction is necessary in unstable patella since delayed primary repair of the MPFL after primary patella dislocation does not reduce the risk of redislocation.[1] The achievement of correct ligament tension in the MPFL reconstruction is extremely important. Therefore, overtightening of the graft is to be avoided. If the MPFL reconstruction is done first, the performance of the ligament after a distal realignment can be easily modified. Thus, it must always be the last step in the procedure.

To reconstruct the MPFL, the authors' preferred graft is the ipsilateral *gracilis tendon* (GT), as it is long and strong enough to duplicate the MPFL function.[4,6] Additional advantages are little harvest-site morbidity, minor alterations of hamstrings' function as well as the easy passage through the patellar bone drill holes. The GT can be easily seen by dissecting the *pes anserinus* bursa and opening the *sartorius* fascia on its upper half. The GT is then exposed and released with a tendon stripper. A whipstitch suture is performed on each end of the tendon with No. 0 high-resistance nonabsorbable sutures. The tendon is sized by using a set of regular anterior cruciate ligament tunnel sizers, and it is then stored within a moist swab. Later, a 2 cm vertical skin incision is made over the superior medial border of the patella to expose its proximal one third. This area corresponds to the MPFL anatomical origin. According to the GT size, usually 3–4 mm, two convergent drill holes of approximately 10 mm in depth are created leaving a bone bridge of 7–10 mm. Therefore, a V-shaped tunnel is obtained so that the graft forms a loop through the patella. This tunnel is further enlarged and smoothed with the help of a curved mosquito clamp to make posterior tendon passage easier. After this, a suture passer or a lasso loop is used to leave a suture in place. This suture will later be used to pull the graft through the patellar tunnel.

Thereon, another 2–3 cm vertical skin approach is made near the medial femoral epicondyle, where the MPFL has its femoral attachment. The femoral attachment of the MPFL has been localized at a point 10 mm distal to the *adductor tubercle* and posterosuperior to the medial epicondyle.[10] It has fibres spreading proximally toward the *adductor tubercle* and distally toward the superficial medial collateral ligament.[7] Therefore, an area between the medial epicondyle and *adductor tubercle* is considered optimal for reconstruction.[14] In the authors' technique, the hiatus of the *adductor magnus* tendon is instead used as a post for the graft. The use of the *adductor's magnus* as a post for MPFL medial attachment is obviously a variation of the anatomical insertion point of this ligament. However, this position has recently been demonstrated to have quasi-isometric behaviur[9] that does not cause significant changes to the patellofemoral contact pressures with respect to an anatomical reconstruction.[5]

After dissecting the tendon of the *adductor magnus*, another provisional loop suture is made around it as a passer for the graft. Then, a subfascial dissection between both the epicondylar and parapatellar incisions is done with the help of a curved blunt forceps in order to make the pathway for the new ligament.[16] At this point, the graft is first passed through the patella leaving an asymmetrical length at both ends. Next, a loop around the *adductor magnus* tendon with the longer limb of the graft is used to again pass it back through the same subfascial via to the patellar attachment. The knee is cycled several times through full range of motion while keeping the graft under tension. In this way, the graft is prestretched and finally it is sutured at 30° of flexion with some No. 0 high-resistance nonabsorbable sutures so that the patella tilt can be manually lateralized 10 mm. It is important not to over constrain the final construct, which would create a patellar chondral overload in flexion[8] or an extensor lag if it is too tight in extension.[15] Additionally, if the graft is long enough, the remaining tendon can be fixed onto the anterior part of the patella by subperiosteally dissecting the extensor mechanism at this level. It is done in order to avoid a larger bone tunnel thus diminishing the risk of joint penetration or patellar fracture. The wounds are closed in the usual way and once the procedure has finished, the patient is left in a brace locked in full extension.

Further advantages of this procedure are that the MPFL reconstruction turns into a simple soft tissue procedure in which the femoral physeal line is not violated as no tunnel is drilled and no hardware is used to fix the graft to the bone. For this reason, the same technique can also be used in skeletally immature patients, since drilling holes through the physis at the femoral epicondyle is no longer necessary.

4.4 Postoperative Management

For the first 2 weeks, patients' knees are maintained in full extension with a knee brace. Full weight bearing with crutches is allowed from the beginning as tolerated. Thereafter, the brace is discontinued. At week 6, knee flexion at 90° is the target. After week 6, free low-demand activities are allowed. Sport-specific drills may be started and gradually progressed after 3 months. Full activity and a return to contact sports may begin 6 months after surgery.

4.5 Summary

This chapter describes a combined distal extensor realignment as well as MPFL reconstruction procedure using a hamstring tendon for chronic patellar instability. Although several predisposing factors are involved in lateral patellar dislocation, the authors believe that the MPFL plays a crucial role as a primary restraint among the medial patellar stabilizers. In this chapter, the detailed surgical technique and the rationale for its reconstruction are presented.

References

1. Christiansen S, Jakobsen B, Lund B, et al. Repair of the medial patellofemoral ligament in primary dislocation of the patella: a prospective randomized study. Arthroscopy. 2008;24:881-7.
2. Fulkerson JP. Anteromedialization of the tibial tuberosity for patellofemoral malalignment. Clin Orthop Relat Res. 1983;177:176-81.

3. Fulkerson JP, Becker GJ, Meaney JA, et al. Anteromedial tibial tubercle transfer without bone graft. Am J Sports Med. 1990;18:490-6.

4. Hamner DL, Brown CH Jr, Steiner ME, et al. Hamstring tendon grafts for reconstruction of the ACL: biomechanical evaluation of the use of multiple strands and tensioning techniques. J Bone Joint Surg. 1999;81-A:549-57.

5. Melegari T, Parks B, Matthews L. Patellofemoral contact area and pressure after medial patellofemoral ligament reconstruction. Am J Sports Med. 2008;36:747-52.

6. Mountney J, Senavongse W, Amis A, et al. Tensile strength of the medial patellofemoral ligament before and after repair or reconstruction. J Bone Joint Surg. 2005;87-B:36-40.

7. Nomura E, Inoue M, Osada N. Anatomical analysis of the medial patellofemoral ligament of the knee, especially the femoral attachment. Knee Surg Sports Traumatol Arthrosc. 2005;13:510-5.

8. Ostermeier S, Holst M, Bohnsack M, et al. In vitro kinematics following reconstruction of the medial patellofemoral ligament. Knee Surg Sports Traumatol Arthrosc. 2007;15:276-85.

9. Panagopoulos A, van Niekerk L, Triantafillopoulos IK. MPFL reconstruction for recurrent patella dislocation: a new surgical technique and review of the literature. Int J Sports Med. 2008;29:359-65.

10. Phillippot R, Chouteau J, Wegrzyn J, et al. Medial patellofemoral ligament anatomy: implications for its surgical reconstruction. Knee Surg Sports Traumatol Arthrosc. 2009;17:475-9.

11. Redziniak D, Diduch D, Mihalko W, et al. Patellar instability. J Bone Joint Surg. 2009;91-A:2264-75.

12. Sallay PI, Poggi J, Speer KP, et al. Acute dislocation of the patella; a correlative pathoanatomic study. Am J Sports Med. 1996;24:52-60.

13. Schöttle P, Fucentese S, Romero J. Clinical and radiological outcome of medial patellofemoral ligament reconstruction with a semitendinosus autograft for patella instability. Knee Surg Sports Traumatol Arthrosc. 2005;13:516-21.

14. Smirk C, Morris H. The anatomy and reconstruction of the patellofemoral ligament. Knee. 2003;10:221-7.

15. Thaunat M, Erasmus P. Management of overtight medial patellofemoral ligament reconstruction. Knee Surg Sports Traumatol Arthrosc. 2009;17:480-3.

16. Warren L, Marshall J. The supporting and layers on the medial side of the knee. J Bone Joint Surg. 1979;61-A:56-62.

Chapter 5
Reconstruction of the Lateral Patellofemoral Ligament: How I Do It

Jack T. Andrish

5.1 Introduction

Ostensibly, reconstruction of the lateral patellofemoral ligament should be used for the treatment of medial instability of the patella.[1,6,7,15] And that it should. But in my hands, a far more frequent use of this lateral reconstruction is for the surgical reconstruction of the extensor mechanism of knee after having failed prior surgery for the treatment of *lateral* instability of the patella when a lateral retinacular release had been included in the procedure. The relative contributions of the lateral retinaculum to medial and lateral patellar stability have been well described.[3,8,12] But in brief, the lateral retinaculum contributes not only to medial restraint of the patella, but lateral restraint as well. Perhaps it is best if we remember to visualize the lateral retinaculum as exerting a sagittal force upon the patella that helps to engage and hold the patella within the femoral trochlea, rather than a predominantly horizontal force that would be implied from most illustrations.

J.T. Andrish
Department of Orthopaedic Surgery,
Center of Sports Health, Cleveland Clinic,
Cleveland, OH, USA
e-mail: andrisj@ccf.org

V. Sanchis-Alfonso (ed.), *Patellar Instability Surgery in Clinical Practice,* DOI 10.1007/978-1-4471-4501-1_5,
© Springer-Verlag London 2013

47

Medial subluxation and even dislocation of the patella is a disabling condition, almost exclusively produced by an enthusiastic lateral retinacular release, often in the face of native pathoanatomies such as trochlear dysplasia or the iatrogenic pathoanatomy of a medialization of the tibial tuberosity.[10] As Fulkerson described, the hallmark of medial patellar instability is the patient that experiences pain and dysfunction out of proportion to what they were experiencing before their surgery for lateral instability.[4] That said, the objective documentation and criteria used to diagnose medial instability of the patella has not been uniform.[11] Most measures use clinical tests that elicit pain and apprehension or abnormal hypermobility of the patella. Others use radiographic demonstrations of increased medial translation under stress or kinematic demonstrations with MRI of excessive medial movement and position.[13,16] I have preferred to use the "relocation test" described by Fulkerson as an indicator of medial patellar subluxation as a cause of the patient's pain, "locking," and giving-way.[4]

5.2   Indications

I have three indications for lateral reconstruction of the patellar retinaculum: (1) symptomatic medial instability of the patella following lateral retinacular release, (2) failed prior surgery for lateral instability of the patella wherein a lateral retinacular release had been included, and (3) multidirectional instability of the patella, sometimes following failed prior surgery and sometimes associated with hyperelasticity syndromes such as Ehlers–Danlos Syndrome.

I cannot emphasize enough the importance and contribution to patellar stability, both medial and lateral, that is played by the lateral retinaculum. As Larson described many years ago, it is better to lengthen the lateral retinaculum rather than release, especially when treating patellar instability.[9] And when performing revision surgery for patellar instability, remember to check for competence of the lateral retinaculum and reconstruct if necessary.

5.3   Contraindications

If for some reason the iliotibial band has been violated and used during prior surgery, then we should look for alternative methods of reconstruction, or even repair. If the patellar instability were also associated with lateral or posterolateral instability of the knee, I would not violate the integrity of the iliotibial band.

5.4   Surgical Technique

The purpose of this technique is to reconstruct the deep transverse layer of the lateral retinaculum and *not* technically, the lateral patellofemoral ligament. Amis has described the lateral retinaculum and noted that the true lateral patellofemoral ligaments are thickenings of the lateral capsule.[2] There is a lateral epicondylopatellar ligament described and present in some individuals, to a varying degree of frequency, but the superficial oblique and deep transverse retinacular layers are more consistent.[5,14] The superficial oblique retinaculum is quite thin. The deep transverse retinaculum is stout, oriented in an optimal direction to restrain the patella, and attached to the lateral boarder of the patella and the deep surface of the iliotibial band. To date, we do not have studies that document the relative contributions of these *individual components* of the lateral retinaculum and lateral capsule to patellar stability.[2] That said, I have chosen to try to reconstruct what appears to be the layer most suited to restrain the patella, the deep transverse lateral retinaculum.

1. The surgical incision is often dictated by the location of prior incisions, but my preferred incision is located anterolateral. It begins 2 cm proximal to the superolateral border of the patella and extends distally to the level of, and just anterior to, Gurdy's tubercle.

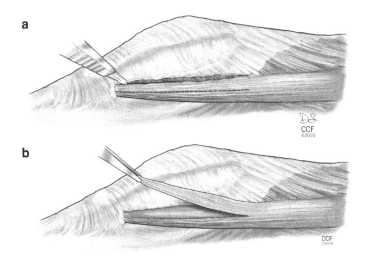

FIGURE 5.1 The lateral retinaculum is exposed to include the iliotibial band (**a**). The anterior half of the iliotibial band is detached from Gurdy's tubercle and then reflected proximally, beyond the lateral femoral epicondyle (**b**) (Copyright The Cleveland Clinic Foundation)

2. Dissection is then carried posterior to expose what is left of the lateral retinaculum and onward to expose the iliotibial band. I then will isolate the anterior half of the iliotibial band (about 1.5 cm in width) and detach this portion from its insertion onto Gurdy's tubercle (Fig. 5.1a). This strip is then reflected proximally well beyond the level of the lateral femoral epicondyle (Fig. 5.1b).
3. Often, there is only a thin layer present that represents the lateral capsule and the scar remains of the lateral retinaculum. In that case, the iliotibial band transfer is laid directly over this tissue. But if there is some manner of (superficial oblique) retinaculum present, then an interval is developed deep to this tissue and superficial to the capsule (Fig. 5.2a). The isolated strip of iliotibial band is brought forth between these layers in order to be attached to the lateral border of the patella (Fig. 5.2b).

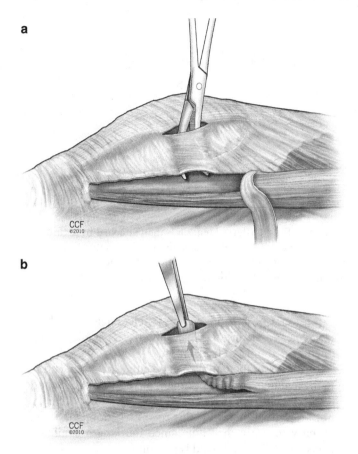

FIGURE 5.2 If there is some manner of attenuated lateral retinaculum remaining, an interval is developed between the lateral capsule and the retinaculum (**a**). The strip of iliotibial band is then brought through this interval to be attached to the lateral border of the junction of the middle and proximal third of the patella (**b**) (Copyright The Cleveland Clinic Foundation)

4. When attaching and tensioning this tendon transfer, I prefer to have a bolster beneath the knee to position the knee in about 20° of flexion. Although it could be debated about the biomechanical advisability of flexion versus

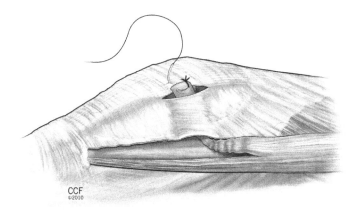

FIGURE 5.3 The transferred tendon is then attached by suture to the remaining peripatellar retinacular tissue, or by suture anchor. It is not necessary to attempt attachment by a drill hole (Copyright The Cleveland Clinic Foundation)

extension, I prefer to have the patella engaged within the trochlea as a means of preventing overtensioning and producing an abnormal translation.

5. Attachment to the patella can be either by direct suture to the remaining pre and peripatellar retinaculum if there is adequate tissue present, or by suture anchor (Fig. 5.3). I do not prefer drill holes for this reconstruction, nor would it be easy to use a drill hole since the length available of transferred iliotibial band is just sufficient to reach the lateral border of the patella.

6. At this point, the orientation of the transferred iliotibial band is somewhat oblique to the patella. Our goal is to make it transversely oriented and "attached" to the remaining iliotibial band at the level of the lateral femoral epicondyle. In order to do this, and to adjust and establish tension, I begin a series of sutures reattaching the posterior border of the transferred tendon to the anterior border of the remaining intact iliotibial band. This begins at the proximal location of the isolation and works distally

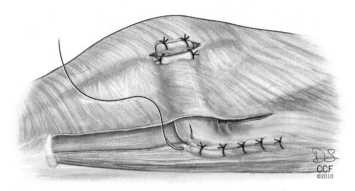

FIGURE 5.4 Our goal is to make the transferred tendon transversely oriented and "attached" to the remaining intact iliotibial band at the level of the lateral femoral epicondyle. In order to do this, and to adjust and establish tension, a series of sutures are placed reattaching the posterior border of the transferred tendon to the anterior border of the remaining intact iliotibial band. This begins at the proximal location of the isolation and works distally until the desired orientation and tension of the transfer has been achieved (Copyright The Cleveland Clinic Foundation)

until the desired orientation and tension of the transfer has been achieved. Simple sutures work well (Fig. 5.4).

7. Often, there will appear to be a kink or wrinkle at the anterior bend of the transfer. In this case, I will place one additional suture within this fold and attach to either itself or the posterior border of the remaining lateral retinaculum to "un-kink" the fold (Fig. 5.5a, b).

8. If there is native lateral retinaculum present, then it is repaired to the lateral border of the patella, if possible, and even at times to the remaining intact iliotibial band. The deep transverse retinaculum has now been reconstructed deep to the remnants of lateral retinaculum.

9. The knee is passed through a range of motion from full extension to at least 90° of flexion to judge patellar tracking and to observe the competence of the suture attachments.

10. Wound closure is routine.

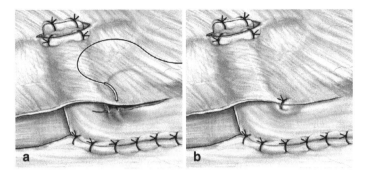

Figure 5.5 Often, there will be a kink at the bend of the transfer. A simple suture from the corner of the iliotibial band to remaining retinacular tissue improves the alignment (**a**). All sutures in place and properly "tensioned," the deep transverse lateral retinaculum has been reconstructed (**b**) (Copyright The Cleveland Clinic Foundation)

5.5   Postoperative Management

Since most often I use this procedure as a part of a revision surgery for lateral or multidirectional patellar instability, the postoperative care is directed by the aggregate of what was done. But for an isolated lateral reconstruction, I apply a cooling unit over an elastic dressing and then apply a double upright brace with a motion control hinge set to allow full extension but block flexion at 40°. The procedure is performed as an outpatient and the dressing left in place until their first return to the office at 1 week. No drains are used. Upon the first return, the dressing is removed and the patient is instructed to use the brace only at nighttime and for community ambulation to "protect" against the odd fall. They are advised to ambulate with the use of crutches with full weight bearing as tolerated. But out of the brace, they are encouraged to move the knee as tolerated without limits. Physical therapy is begun at this time, out of the brace, for range of motion exercises and pelvifemoral conditioning. The subcuticular sutures are removed at 3 weeks and the average length of time needed for crutch support is 3–6 weeks.

5.6   Pearls and Pitfalls

Don't forget the importance of a competent lateral retinaculum when dealing with the surgical management of patellar instability. In the first case when performing patellar realignment and reconstructive surgery for patellar instability, it is always safer to lengthen rather than release the lateral retinaculum. And most certainly, never release the lateral retinaculum in the face of trochlear dysplasia, patella alta, or hyperelasticity. In the case of revision surgery for failed patellar realignment and reconstruction, do not forget to establish a competent lateral retinaculum, even if the only observable instability is lateral. Although not common, I have had cases of recurrent lateral patellar subluxations where the only technique required to correct the problem was a lateral reconstruction alone, not medial. It is amazing.

And what is my biggest pitfall? Making the wrong diagnosis of medial patellar instability as the primary cause of the patient's pain and mechanical symptoms. Many if not most of the patients with symptomatic iatrogenic medial patellar instability have *chronic* pain and chronic pain is multifactorial with a different pathoneurophysiology than acute pain. The mere fact that the patient can subluxate and even dislocate their patella medially is no guarantee that their pain and disability are directly due to the instability. Go with caution into that dark night.

5.7   Clinical Results and Complications

Since most of the patients that have this procedure have multiple mechanical and, at times, psychosocial issues involved, the clinical results cannot be isolated to the lateral reconstruction alone. My "results" of those patients with only an isolated lateral reconstruction are therefore anecdotal. I can say, however, that I have been using this technique for over 15 years and continue to use it as my primary method of lateral reconstruction. Complications and poor results, as related above, are mostly a product of misinterpreting and misunderstanding the multifactorial pathology involved in the patient.

References

1. Abhaykumar S, Craig DM. Fascia lata sling reconstruction for recurrent medical dislocation of the patella. Knee. 1999;6:55-7.
2. Amis A. Current concepts on anatomy and biomechanics of patellar stability. Sports Med Arthrosc. 2007;15:48-56.
3. Desio SM, Burks RT, Bachus K. Soft tissue restraints to lateral patellar translation in the human knee. Am J Sports Med. 1998;26:59-65.
4. Fulkerson J. Anterolateralization of the tibial tubercle. Tech Orthop. 1997;12:165-9.
5. Fulkerson J, Gossling H. Anatomy of the knee joint lateral retinaculum. Clin Orthop Relat Res. 1980;153:183-8.
6. Hughston J, Deese M. Medial subluxation of the patella as a complication of lateral retinacular release. Am J Sports Med. 1988;16:383-8.
7. Hughston J, Flandry F, Brinker M, et al. Surgical correction of medial subluxation of the patella. Am J Sports Med. 1996;24:486-93.
8. Ishibashi Y, Okamura Y, Otsuka H, et al. Lateral patellar retinaculum tension in patellar instability. Clin Orthop Relat Res. 2002;397: 362-9.
9. Larson R, Cabaud HE, Slocum D, et al. The patellar compression syndrome: surgical treatment by lateral retinacular release. Clin Orthop Relat Res. 1978;134:158-67.
10. Metcalf R. An arthroscopic method for lateral release of the subluxating or dislocating patella. Clin Orthop Relat Res. 1982;167:9-18.
11. Nonweiler DE, DeLee JC. The diagnosis and treatment of medial subluxation of the patella after lateral retinacular release. Am J Sports Med. 1994;22:680-6.
12. Senavongse W, Farahmand F, Jones J, et al. Quantitative measurement of patellofemoral joint stability: force-displacement behavior of the human patella in vitro. J Orthop Res. 2003;21:780-6.
13. Shellock F, Mink J, Deutsch A, et al. Evaluation of patients with persistent symptoms after lateral retinacular release by kinematic magnetic resonance imaging of the patellofemoral joint. Arthroscopy. 1990;6:226-34.
14. Starok M, Lenchik L, Trudell D, et al. Normal patellar retinaculum: MR and sonographic imaging with cadaveric correlation. AJR. 1997;168:1493-9.
15. Teitge R, Spak R. Lateral patellofemoral ligament reconstruction. Arthroscopy. 2004;20:998-1002.
16. Teitge R, Faerber W, Des Madryl P, et al. Stress radiographs of the patellofemoral joint. J Bone Joint Surg. 1996;78-A:193-203.

Chapter 6
Reconstruction of the Lateral Patellofemoral Ligament: How I Do It

Robert A. Teitge and Roger Torga-Spak

6.1 Introduction

Medial dislocation or subluxation of the patella is a disabling condition that can occur after an isolated lateral release, or after lateral release in combination with tibial tubercle transfer or medial soft tissue imbrications.[2-4,6-8]

Techniques to repair the lateral retinaculum can be found in the literature,[5,6] as well as descriptions of reconstruction with local soft-tissue augmentation (fascia lata, patellar tendon).[1,4] In our experience with lateral retinacular repair and imbrication, a noticeable increase in medial excursion usually would reappear after the first postoperative year. This led us to develop a technique for lateral patellofemoral ligament (LPFL) reconstruction following the same principles of the medial patellofemoral ligament reconstruction previously described: (1) selection of a sufficiently strong and stiff graft, (2) isometric graft placement, (3) adequate fixation, (4) correct tension, and (5) no condylar rubbing or impingement.

R. Torga-Spak (✉)
Faculty of Orthopaedics and Traumatology
Department of Surgery, Instituto Universitario CEMIC,
Buenos Aires, Argentina
e-mail: rogerts@traumatologiapenta.com.ar

V. Sanchis-Alfonso (ed.), *Patellar Instability Surgery in Clinical Practice,* DOI 10.1007/978-1-4471-4501-1_6,
© Springer-Verlag London 2013

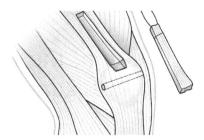

FIGURE 6.1 Harvesting of the quadriceps graft. A transversal tunnel is performed through the patella

6.2 Surgical Technique

6.2.1 Graft Selection and Harvesting

The quadriceps tendon provides a reliable graft but bone–patellar tendon–bone and Achilles allograft can also be used. With the knee in extension, a 6- to 8-cm skin incision is made midway between the lateral epicondyle and the lateral edge of the patella. A 4- to 5-mm × 1-cm partial-thickness quadriceps tendon is obtained. The posterior quadriceps tendon is left intact to avoid scar in the synovial pouch. A 1 cm² × 5-mm thick bone is removed from the superior central one third of the patella with a small oscillating saw. The graft is harvested from the quadriceps tendon, as far proximal as feasible, and generally 8–10 cm can be obtained before the muscle fibers of the vastus lateralis and vastus medialis converge (Fig. 6.1). The graft is prepared by drilling a 2.5-mm hole through the bone block and then running a No. 2 Vicryl suture from the free tendon end toward the bone block and back using the Krackow technique.

6.2.2 Isometric Location

The graft must be located isometrically to avoid overstretching it to failure during joint motion or to avoid overconstraining

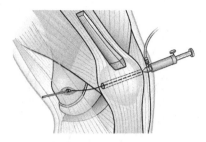

FIGURE 6.2 Isometric location of the insertion point in the lateral condyle

patellar motion. A transverse 2.5-mm hole is placed through the patella at about the mid one third height. A strand of No. 2 Vicryl is passed through this hole and a small loop tied on the lateral aspect. A 2.5-mm K-wire is placed through this loop and into the bone of the lateral femoral condyle at about the position of the lateral epicondyle. Next, the pneumatic Isometer is inserted into the hole in the medial patella and the No. 2 Vicryl isometric measurement suture passed into it (Fig. 6.2). The knee is then placed through a full range of motion while the change in length of the lateral suture is read in the Isometer. Adjustments in the position of the K-wire in the lateral condyle are made until no excursion is read in the isometer during the full range of motion.

6.2.3   Secure Fixation

The bone block is countersunk into the femur and fixed with a 4.0-mm fully threaded lag screw. To create an accurate countersunk hole for the bone block in the femur, the bone block that has the 2.5-mm diameter hole in it is slid over the K-wire, which locates the isometric site on the femur. Then the bone block lies against the femur like a template while a thin chisel outlines the bone block and penetrates the cortex of the lateral femoral condyle. Because the femoral bone is often osteoporotic from disuse, cancellous bone is impacted instead of removed to create the recess for the

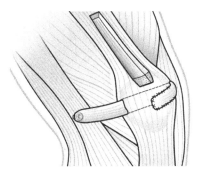

FIGURE 6.3 Quadriceps graft fixed to the lateral condyle, passed through the patellar tunnel, and sutured on the anterior aspect of the patella

patellar bone block. It is then fixed with a 4.0-mm lag screw. An adequate bone tunnel can be placed transversely through the patella with two parallel 4.5- to 6-mm drills, avoiding the anterior tension trabeculae in the patella and avoiding the articular surface. Fixation of the quadriceps tendon to the patella is easily accomplished by pulling the tendon graft into the oval transverse tunnel in the patella, out the medial side, and turning it superficially onto the anterior surface of the patella, where it is sutured to the quadriceps expansion (Fig. 6.3).

6.2.4   Correct Tension

The tension set in the graft must be enough to limit medial excursion to an amount that approximates that of the normal contralateral knee. We set the tension with the knee flexed 60°–90° to avoid the risk of pulling too far lateral. Do not set the tension with the patella outside the trochlea. Realize that the ligament is not a dynamic structure that pulls the patella laterally, but rather a static restraint that holds the patella against moving too far medially.

6.2.5   Avoid Impingement

When the correct location is found, the patellar bone block is countersunk into the femur to avoid a prominence producing an iliotibial band friction syndrome. The range of motion must be tested to ensure there is no restriction of patellar or knee motion. The graft should not be rubbing against the lateral femoral condyle. If impingement on the wall of the lateral femoral condyle is detected, the graft can be placed on the anterior surface of the patella and pulled into the medial tunnel in a lateral direction.

6.3   Postoperative Care

Postoperative treatment is to allow full range of motion, full weight bearing, continuous passive motion, active exercises, but avoiding stairs, squatting, and resistive leg extension until the patellar bone donor site has adequate time to heal.

6.4   Our Experience

This procedure has been performed in our institution since 1980 in 80 patients. The results have been excellent when assessed from stability standpoint and none of the knees has lost the stability obtained at surgery. Three patients have sustained a patellar fracture, which occurred with a fall in the early postoperative phase; two of them have required open reduction and internal fixation. This is a salvage procedure for repair of medial iatrogenic instability. It does not address the original source of complaint. It clearly cannot improve or reverse osteoarthrosis, chondromalacia, bony malalignment, or lateral instability caused by an insufficient medial patellofemoral ligament.

In cases with associated medial and lateral patellar instability (multidirectional instability) a combination of the techniques described to reconstruct the MPFL and LPFL can be used.

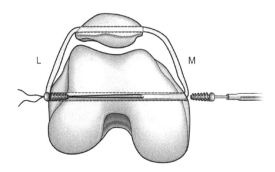

FIGURE 6.4 Combined MPFL and LPFL reconstruction passing a free graft through a transverse patellar and epicondylar tunnel

An option for reconstruction of both patellofemoral ligaments during the same procedure is by means of a free semitendinosus graft passed through a transverse patellar and transepicondylar tunnel (Fig. 6.4).

References

1. Abhaykumar S, Craig DM. Fascia Lata sling reconstruction for recurrent medial dislocation of the patella. Knee. 1999;6:55-7.
2. Blazina NE. Complications of the Hauser procedure. In: Kennedy JC, editor The injured adolescent knee. Baltimore: Williams & Wilkins; 1979. p. 198.
3. Eppley RA. Medial patellar subluxation. In: Fox JM, Del Pizzo W, editors The patellofemoral joint. New York: McGraw Hill; 1993:149-56.
4. Hughston JC, Deese M. Medial subluxation of the patella as a complication of lateral retinacular release. Am J Sports Med. 1988;16:383-8.
5. Johnson DP, Wakeley C. Reconstruction of the lateral patellar retinaculum following lateral release: a case report. Knee Surg Sports Traumatol Arthrosc. 2002;10:361-3.
6. Nonweiler DE, DeLee JC. The diagnosis and treatment of medial subluxation of the patella after lateral retinacular release. Am J Sports Med. 1994;22:680-6.

7. Shea KP, Fulkerson JP. Preoperative computed tomography scanning and arthroscopy in predicting outcome after lateral retinacular release. Arthroscopy. 1992;8:327-34.
8. Small NC. An analysis of complications in lateral retinacular release procedures. Arthroscopy. 1989;15:282-6.

Chapter 7
Osteotomies Around the Patellofemoral Joint

Roland M. Biedert and Philippe M. Tscholl

7.1 Introduction

A normal patellofemoral gliding mechanism with perfect stability is guaranteed by the complex interaction of skeletal geometry, soft tissues, and neuromuscular control.[10] During knee flexion, the patella moves from a medial to a lateral tilted position as knee flexion approaches 90°.[29,32,33,51,53] Abnormal skeletal geometry – such as increased femoral anteversion, trochlear dysplasia, patella alta or infera, increased tibial external torsion, increased tibial tubercle lateralization, and variations of combined deformities – may lead to patellofemoral complaints.[10] Altered vectors and forces acting on the patellofemoral joint (PFJ) can cause cartilage failure with secondary osteoarthritis instability and musculotendinous insufficiency. Osteotomy with soft tissue balancing might be the best treatment, depending on the underlying pathology. Surgery aims to eliminate the present pathomorphology.

R.M. Biedert (✉)
Sportclinic Villa Linde, Swiss Olympic Medical Center
Magglingen-Biel, University of Basel, Biel, Switzerland
e-mail: r.biedert@bluewin.ch

V. Sanchis-Alfonso (ed.), *Patellar Instability Surgery in Clinical Practice*, DOI 10.1007/978-1-4471-4501-1_7,
© Springer-Verlag London 2013

7.2   Femur

7.2.1   Pathologic Femoral Anteversion

Patient's complaints may appear as a diffuse knee or hip pain and even present with patellar dislocation in some cases. Others may be asymptomatic; however are bothered by the appearance of their leg axes. Typically it begins at the young age, although some may be up to 50 years of age at the onset of symptoms.

Since increased femoral anteversion (coxa antetorta) is most frequent, decreased femoral anteversion (coxa retro-torta) is not further described in this section.

7.2.1.1   Physical Examination

In *supine* position, increased internal rotation of the distal femoral head is apparent with both knee caps verged inter-nal, also known as "squinting patellae".[48] Examination of hip rotation in 90° flexion shows increased internal rotation com-pared to the external rotation, and may reach up to 80–90°.[16] Physical examination of the patella highlights an often tilted and rarely lateralized position. Tender points are found along the lateral patellar facet due to hypercompression on the lateral trochlea, potential soft tissue impingement, and pain-ful lateral retinaculum.

In the *sitting* position with hanging lower extremity, the patella is well centered (with mild negative lateral patellar tilt) in the trochlear groove, and therefore the tuberculum–sulcus angle is normal.

When *standing* in a comfortable position, the feet are slightly externally rotated (10–15°), but the patellae are internally rotated on the distal femur (Fig. 7.1a). Active correction of the patella position to normal (straight to anterior) causes increased and no more comfortable external rotation of the feet (Fig. 7.1b). In some patients, coxa saltans may be seen, when the iliotibial tract skips over the greater trochanter. Additional clinical findings, such as the too many toes sign, may be observed.

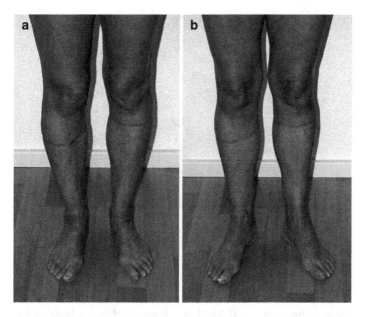

FIGURE 7.1 (**a**) Internally rotated patellae in comfortable standing position. (**b**) Active correction of the patella to normal causes increased external rotation of the feet

7.2.1.2   Imaging

CT Evaluation

Lower extremity alignment is measured by series of 2D-CT scans. The following planes are selected: greater trochanter, distal femur, tibial head, and malleolus. Greater trochanter and distal femur are superimposed, and the angle of the femoral anteversion is measured (Fig. 7.2). Values of more than 20° are considered as pathologic.[10,39] At the same time, tibial rotation and TT-TG distance should be analyzed, since concomitant findings are frequent and crucial for successful therapy.[24]

Any other causes of patellar maltracking and its subsequent damage should be eliminated.

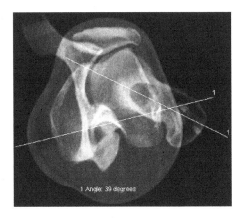

FIGURE 7.2 Axial CT evaluation of the femoral anteversion. The femoral anteversion is 39°

Plain Radiographs and MRI

Plain radiographs and MRI are demanded to exclude other pathologies, such as cartilage lesions and trochlear dysplasia.

7.2.1.3 Special Considerations

For practical understanding it is crucial to know that the underlying cause is not a malpositioning of the patella; it is a malrotation of the distal femur with regard to the knee extensor mechanism alignment.

Muscular causes, such as insufficiency or contractures, need to be ruled out. Malalignment of the tibia or biomechanical failures such as hyperpronation of the foot may clinically mimic increased femoral anteversion or may concomitantly exist described as "miserable malalignment syndrome" by James et al.[37]

Often, a tight lateral retinaculum is preexisting, and therefore soft tissue balancing should be considered in surgical therapy.

7.2.1.4   Conservative Treatment

Conservative approach represents the first-line treatment with enforcing external hip rotators, stretching of the internal rotators and of the lateral retinaculum. Cofindings such as hyperpronation of the foot, which causes more internal femoral rotation, may be corrected by insoles. Usually, conservative treatment does not relieve pain sufficiently, especially in younger patients. In elderly patient, retropatellar osteoarthritis on the lateral patellar facet and/or lateral trochlea may appear.

7.2.1.5   Surgery

The surgical treatment with rotational femur osteotomy may be performed on the intertrochanteric or supracondylar level. The authors prefer the distal femoral correction, especially when additional interventions are necessary in the knee joint at the same time.[10] The correctional procedure on the intertrochanteric level is therefore not further discussed. The physis must be closed completely.

Supracondylar Rotation Osteotomy

Lateral incision from the lateral epicondylus of the knee is chosen for posterolateral approach to the femur. The vastus lateralis and intermedius muscles are delaminated from the lateral supracondylar line.[35] Three to five centimeter above the metaphysis, two Kirschner wires are placed to monitor both the present and the desired rotation after correction (Fig. 7.3). Always protecting the medial neurovascular bundle, the osteotomy is performed horizontally. The two Kirschner wires are rotated as the preoperative planning based on what the CT assessment has indicated. Fixation of the osteotomy is performed by locking screw osteosynthesis plate, which has at least three distal and three proximal bicortical screws for fixation (Fig. 7.4). Patellar soft tissue balancing with lengthening of the lateral retinaculum and shortening

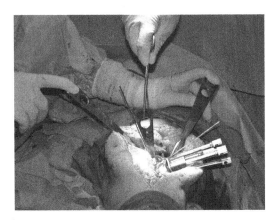

FIGURE 7.3 Two Kirschner wires indicate the angle of correction

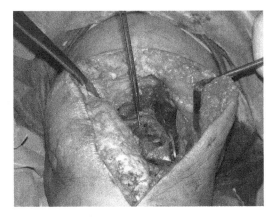

FIGURE 7.4 Fixation of the supracondylar rotation osteotomy

of the medial patellofemoral ligament is done at the end, if needed. Closure is performed layer by layer of the soft tissues and preventing potential muscular hernia.

7.2.1.6   Postoperative Rehabilitation

Mobilization is initiated the first day after surgery with partial weight bearing of 10 kg for 6 weeks. During these first

6 weeks, healing of the osteotomy, decreasing swelling, and activation of quadriceps muscle are the main objectives. Plain radiographs verify after 6 weeks the postoperative healing of the osteotomy. If the consolidation of the osteotomy is correct, full weight bearing can be started immediately. When sufficient mobility has been regained, treadmill exercises can be started (generally 8 week after surgery). No restriction of activities is advised 6 months after osteotomy.

7.2.1.7 Summary

Increased femoral anteversion is a complex biomechanical pathology which frequently includes also malalignments of the tibia and the foot. Surgical treatment with supracondylar osteotomy has shown good results in patients with patellar maltracking symptoms and (sub-)luxation when conservative treatment failed.

7.2.2 Trochlear Dysplasia

The femoral trochlea is important for controlling the patellofemoral gliding mechanism.[7,27] Normal articular shape of trochlea and patella allow for undisturbed patellar tracking. The normal cartilaginous surface of the trochlea consists of the lateral and medial facets of the femoral sulcus and is defined by different criteria in the proximal–distal, medio-lateral, and antero-posterior direction.[10,12,51] The normal trochlea deepens from proximal to distal.[10,51] In the proximal–distal direction, it is longest laterally and shortest on the medial side (Fig. 7.5). The deepened trochlear groove separates the lateral facet from the medial part. In the antero-posterior measurements, the most anterior aspect of the lateral condyle is normally higher than the medial condyle and the deepest point is represented by the center of the trochlear groove.[12]

Trochlear dysplasia is an abnormality of shape and depth of the trochlear groove, mainly in its proximal extent.[19,52]

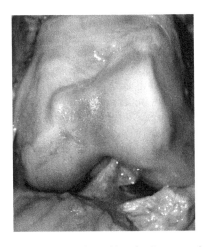

FIGURE 7.5 Shape of a normal trochlea (cadaver study)

It represents an important pathologic articular morphology that is a strong risk factor for permanent patellar instability.[4,7,10,17,19,21-23,26,41,42,50,54,55] Femoral trochlear dysplasia has been reported to occur in up to 85% of patients with recurrent patellar dislocation.[23,55] The trochlear depth may be decreased, the trochlea may be flat, or a trochlear bump is present. According to this, different classifications are described in the literature.[10,17,20] Additionally we found that also a too short lateral trochlea is a frequent cause of proximal–lateral patellar instability and noticed that there exists a widespread variability of combinations of trochlear dysplasia.[8-10,14]

7.2.3   Short Trochlea

7.2.3.1   Physical Examination

The patients with a too short lateral trochlear facet suffer from patellar instability. The patella is well centered in the trochlea under relaxed conditions. But when the patient contracts the quadriceps muscle with the leg in extension, the

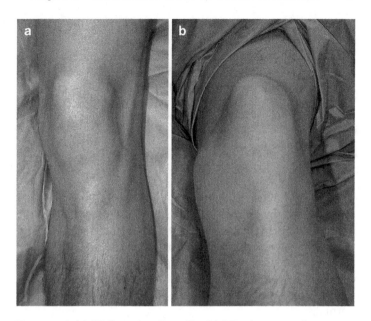

FIGURE 7.6 (**a**) Well-centered patella. (**b**) Muscle contraction causes dynamic superolateral patellar subluxation

patella is pulled to proximal out of the short trochlea because it is no more sufficiently guided and stabilized by the too short lateral facet of the trochlea. In most cases, the contraction causes also subluxation to lateral, a so-called dynamic supero-lateral patellar subluxation (Fig. 7.6a, b). In contrast to the *lateral pull sign*, described by Kolowich et al.[38], this type of patellofemoral instability is primarily not due to soft tissue abnormalities (atrophy of the vastus medialis obliquus and hypertrophy of the vastus lateralis and lateral structures), but caused by a pathologic proximal patellar tracking due to the missing osteochondral opposing force of the lateral trochlear facet. This type of patella instability can also be depicted by manual examination in complete extension of the knee. Only minimal manual pressure to lateral causes the subluxation and discomfort to the patient. In most cases the patient feels pain and tries to resist this manoeuvre. This test in full extension must be differentiated from the *patellar apprehension test* which is performed in 20–30° of knee flexion.[7,45] With increasing knee flexion, the patella enters into the more distal and normal part of the trochlear groove and becomes therefore more and more stable. This confirms the clinical suspicion of proximal lateral patellar instability.

7.2.3.2   Imaging

Radiographs

The radiologic examination of patients with a too short lateral facet of the trochlea do normally not show the typical findings of trochlear dysplasia in the true lateral view such as the crossing sign, supratrochlear spur, double contour[17,19,22,23], or lateral trochlear sign.[31] Radiographs can only show signs of dysplasia in combined trochlear abnormalities.[9,10,14] The different indices used for patellar height measurements are normal.

MR Measurements

MR measurements are performed with the knees in 0° of flexion, the foot in 15° external rotation, and the quadriceps muscle consciously relaxed. Measurements on sagittal images include different parameters.[8,9,14] First, two circles indicate the central longitudinal axis of the femoral shaft (Fig. 7.7). Second, the most lateral sagittal image on which the articular cartilage of the lateral condyle still can be analyzed is selected. A tangent line (d) on the distal femoral cartilage is drawn in 90° degrees to the femoral axis (Ca). The length to the most anterior (A) and the most posterior (P) aspect of the cartilaginous part is measured in relation to the tangent line. Its ratio ([a:p] * 100) represents the lateral condyle index in percentages. The mean lateral condyle index is 93% ± 7 (range 73–109) for patients with normal patellofemoral joints. Therefore we consider an anterior length of the lateral articular facet of the trochlea with index values of 93% or more of the length of the posterior articular cartilage as normal. Index values of less than 90% must

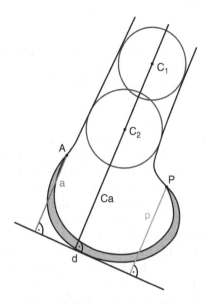

FIGURE 7.7 MR measurements of the lateral condyle index

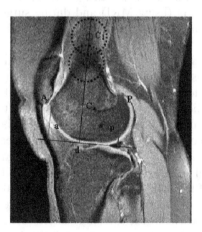

FIGURE 7.8 MR measurement shows a too short lateral condyle index of 75.2%

therefore be considered as pathologic (short) and values of 84% or less confirm the presence of a too short lateral facet (Fig. 7.8).

7.2.3.3   Surgery

Surgical techniques are developed to correct the pathologic morphology. In this situation lengthening is recommended to eliminate the too short lateral trochlea.[10,11,14]

Lengthening

Clear indication for lengthening is given when the lateral condyle index is 84% or less. Lengthening is designed to create a longer proximal part of the lateral trochlear sulcus to improve the contact within the patellofemoral joint and with this to optimize the patellofemoral gliding mechanism. A longer lateral trochlear facet is the feature that must "capture" the patella in extension before the knee starts to flex, to ensure that it is guided into the more distal trochlear groove. Normally, the contact between the articular surface of the trochlea and the articular cartilage behind the patella is about one third of the length of the patellar cartilage (measured using the patellotrochlear index).[11] This value is very helpful both in planning (using MRI) and during surgery to determine how much lengthening to proximal should be performed.

Through a short parapatellar lateral incision the superficial retinaculum is localized. About 1 cm from the border of the patella it is longitudinally incised and carefully separated from the oblique part of the retinaculum in the posterior direction to allow at the end of surgery lengthening of the lateral retinaculum at the same time if needed.[7] Then the oblique part is cut and the patellofemoral joint is opened. The proximal shape of the lateral facet of the trochlea and the length of the articular cartilage are assessed with regard to the length of the sulcus and the medial facet of the trochlea. The presence of a too short lateral articular facet is reconfirmed. In such a case, the patellotrochlear overlap is less than one third. The present overlap allows now to determine the amount of lengthening of the lateral facet and should be about one third at the end, measured in extension (0° of flexion).[7,11] The incomplete lateral osteotomy is made

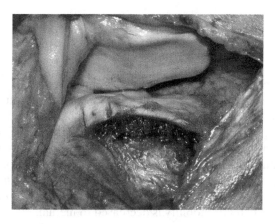

FIGURE 7.9 Lengthening osteotomy

at least 5 mm from the cartilage of the sulcus to prevent necrosis of the trochlea or breaking of the lateral facet. The osteotomy starts at the end of the cartilage (arrow) and is continued approximately 1–1.5 cm to distal into the femoral condyle and to proximal into the femoral shaft, always according to the aimed patellofemoral overlapping. The osteotomy is opened carefully with the use of a chisel. Fracture of the distal cartilage may occur and has no consequences; however sharp edges must be smoothed. Cancellous bone (obtained through a small cortical opening of the lateral condyle more posterior) is inserted and impacted (Fig. 7.9). Additional fixation is possible using resorbable sutures. To finish, the lateral retinaculum is reconstructed in 60° of knee flexion.

7.2.3.4 Postoperative Rehabilitation

The postoperative rehabilitation aims to center the patella in the trochlea, to balance the soft tissue structures, and to strengthen the muscle groups. Partial weight bearing is necessary for 4 weeks. The ROM starts immediately with 0° – 0° – 80° (continuous passive motion included). Full sport activities are possible after 3 months.

7.2.4   Flat Trochlea

7.2.4.1   Physical Examination

The patella is well centered or lateralized with the quadriceps muscle relaxed. Maximum quadriceps contraction pulls the patella to lateral and causes lateral subluxation. In 30° of knee flexion, the patella is less lateralized, but the persisting overhang causes a vacuum effect on the lateral structures. The overhang is caused by tight lateral soft tissues. The apprehension test is positive and painful to lateral, negative to medial. Testing the patellar mobility to lateral, no osseous resistance is noted. Patellar mobility is decreased to medial.[7,10]

7.2.4.2   Imaging

Radiographs

The lateral radiograph shows trochlear dysplasia. The anteroposterior radiograph reveals lateralization of the patella.

Axial CT Evaluation

Axial CT scans confirm trochlear dysplasia. In axial CT scans in 0° extension, the patella is subluxed to the lateral and tilted; the lateral trochlea is flat (Fig. 7.10a).

Quadriceps contraction leads to increased lateral patellar subluxation (Fig. 7.10b). In 30° of knee flexion, the patella is more centered, but still lateralized (caused by the tight lateral structures).

7.2.4.3   Surgery

Conservative treatment is not successful, as it may not influence the structural failure with the trochlear dysplasia. Only surgical treatment may improve the pathomorphology.

Surgery must advise three problems: the flat lateral condyle with the dysplastic trochlea, the tight lateral soft tissues, and the insufficient medial stabilizing structures.[7,10]

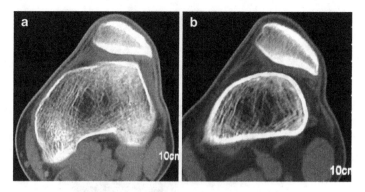

FIGURE 7.10 (**a**) Axial CT scans with flat trochlea and lateralization of the patella (*in extension*). (**b**) Increased lateral subluxation of the patella with muscle contraction (same patient as in Fig.7.10a)

Elevation

The surgical procedure consists of three steps: reconstruction (elevation) of the lateral condyle, lengthening of the lateral structures, and shortening and imbricating of the medial structures.[6,7,10]

Surgery starts with a parapatellar lateral arthrotomy. The flat and the trochlea are inspected. The incomplete lateral osteotomy goes from the proximal edge of the lateral trochlea to distal, always ending proximal to the sulcus terminalis (Fig. 7.11). The osteotomy is opened carefully using a chisel. Fracture of the distal cartilage may occur and has no consequence. Sharp edges must be smoothened. The lateral condyle is then lifted up[1], cancellous bone (taken from the lateral femoral condyle) inserted, and impacted. The amount of raising depends on the form of the trochlea and the femoral condyle. In most cases 5–6 mm are sufficient. Overcorrection must be avoided. Additional fixation is possible using sutures. This reconstruction improves the osseous stability. The last step consists of shortening and imbricating the MPFL and in some cases also the medial retinaculum. The lateral retinacula are adapted in about 50–60° of knee flexion to guarantee lengthening and to eliminate the preoperatively increased

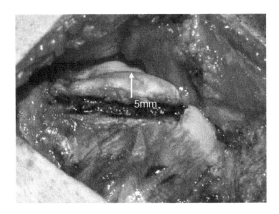

FIGURE 7.11   Intraoperative view after elevation of a flat trochlea

lateral pull. Complications are possible. They include fracturing of the lateral condyle, too much thinning of the osteochondral flap of the lateral trochlea, and loosening of the cancellous bone.

7.2.4.4   Postoperative Rehabilitation

The postoperative rehabilitation aims to center the patella in the trochlea, to balance the soft tissue structures, and to strengthen the muscle groups. Partial weight bearing is necessary for 4 weeks. The ROM starts immediately with $0° – 0° – 80°$ (continuous passive motion included). Full sport activities are possible after 3 months.

7.2.5   Flat and Short Trochlea

Combined pathologies with a too short, but also a flat lateral facet of the trochlea can occur.[8-10,14] This represents another type of trochlear dysplasia causing lateral patellar instability. The surgical steps consist of a lengthening osteotomy with additional elevation of the lateral facet.

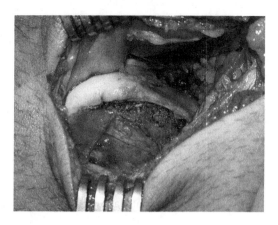

FIGURE 7.12 Lengthening and elevation of a flat and too short trochlea (*right knee*)

7.2.5.1   Lengthening and Elevation

The lateral approach is the same. The osteotomy is opened carefully and the lateral facet lifted up to the desired height and length of the trochlea. The amount of elevation and lengthening depends on the present pathomorphology. The lateral facet of the sulcus should be higher and longer than the medial facet (Fig. 7.12). The anterior cortex of the femoral shaft serves as an orientation of the necessary elevation. In most cases 5–6 mm elevation is sufficient. Overcorrection (with hypercompression) must be strictly avoided. It also has to be considered that in 5 out of 6 cases the lateral condyle is not too flat, but the floor of the trochlea too high.[12] This would be visible on preoperative axial MR images.

7.2.5.2   Postoperative Rehabilitation

Partial weight bearing (10–20 kg) is recommended for 4 weeks to avoid hypercompression of the osteotomy. Range of motion is limited (0°–0°–80°) in the very beginning for some days to decrease swelling and pain. Continuous passive

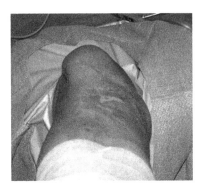

FIGURE 7.13 Subluxation of the patella (*in extension, relaxed*)

motion starts immediately to optimize the patellofemoral gliding mechanism and to form the reconstructed trochlea. Bicycling and swimming are the first allowed sport activities after 2–3 weeks. Sports activities without any restriction are permitted after 3 months.

7.2.6   Central Bump

7.2.6.1   Physical Examination

The patella is spontaneously subluxed to lateral in extension with relaxed muscles (Fig. 7.13). Contraction of the quadriceps muscle may cause complete patellar dislocation. The apprehension test is severely positive to lateral. With increased flexion, the patella moves more medially on the femur. In higher flexion, the apprehension test may become negative and the patella is better stabilized.

7.2.6.2   Imaging

Radiographs

The lateral view shows a severe dysplastic trochlea with crossing sign (Fig. 7.14).[22]

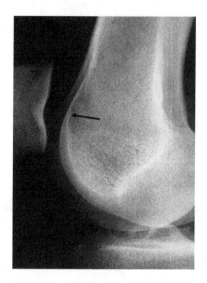

FIGURE 7.14 Crossing sign (*arrow*)

CT Evaluation

Axial CT scans illustrate the convex-shaped dysplastic trochlea with a central bump and the severe lateral subluxation of the patella.[7,55]

MR Measurements

Axial MRI is the best modality to depict the articular shape of the dysplastic trochlea (Fig. 7.15). But the central bump is also visible on sagittal MRI. In addition, cartilage defects on the patella and the femur can be documented.

7.2.6.3   Surgery

The treatment must eliminate the convex-shaped dysplastic trochlea. This provides osseous stability of the patella in the femoral groove, lengthening of the lateral, and doubling of the medial structures.

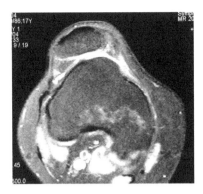

FIGURE 7.15 Central bump with severe patellar subluxation (*axial MRI*)

Deepening Trochleoplasty

This surgical procedure consists of different steps: lengthening of the lateral retinacula, the iliotibial tract, and the vastus lateralis muscle–tendon-unit, doubling of the medial retinaculum and the medial patellofemoral ligament, and deepening of the trochlear groove (trochleoplasty).[3,4,7,19]

The surgical procedure begins with a lateral arthrotomy.[7] The inspection of the joint shows the convex shape of the trochlea with the central bump (Fig. 7.16). The lateral articular part of the trochlea is too short and too flat (even falling off) in reference to the central part. A lateral incision with the knife separates the articular cartilage from the synovial layer. Then the dysplastic trochlea is partially detached from the lateral condyle using a chisel, beginning proximally. The osteochondral flap remains attached distally (Fig. 7.17). It is extremely important not to break the distal attachment. Deepening of the cancellous femoral bone is now performed using a high-speed burr. It is important that the deepening is continued to proximal into the femoral shaft. This guarantees elimination of the central bump.[3] The correct deepening is reached when the new surface is proximally on the same plane as the anterior femoral cortical bone.[19] The detached osteochondral flap of the trochlea is now thinned with a burr

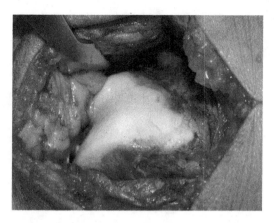

FIGURE 7.16 Convex proximal trochlea with central bump

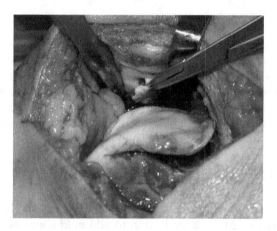

FIGURE 7.17 Osteochondral flap

without removing all bone. Thinning is completed when the osteochondral flap is elastic and fits into the new form of the femur. This step is tested by carefully using a pestle. To keep the osteochondral flap in the new position and to guarantee deepening of the trochlea, the central part of the trochlea is fixed with a resorbable suture (Vicryl 5 mm).[7] Two lateral and two medial resorbable smart nails (length 16 mm) secure the

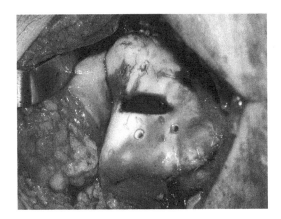

FIGURE 7.18 Deepened trochlea with refixation of the osteochondral flap

reposition of the trochlea. The osteotomy gap is filled with the removed cancellous bone. Single sutures adapt the synovial layer to the articular cartilage (Fig. 7.18). The final step consists of doubling the medial and lengthening the lateral structures.

The risks of this technique include breaking of the osteochondral flap, distal detachment, and too much thinning of the flap, decreasing the blood supply.

7.2.6.4   Postoperative Rehabilitation

Partial weight bearing is recommended for 6 weeks. The knee is placed in 20° of knee flexion to add mild compression to the refixed osteochondral flap. ROM is slowly increased during the first 6 weeks, maximal to 90° of knee flexion. The complete recovery time takes 4–6 months.

7.2.7   Patella Alta

Patella alta is defined as pathologic proximalization of the patella with reference to the tibia or the trochlea.[5,18,30,31,36] The patellofemoral contact surface is decreased in this position and therefore the passive osseous stabilization is low.[13,34] Improvement of patellar stability is noted during flexion. The femur rolls and glides posteriorly on the tibia during knee flexion and the patella glides in accordance into the trochlea.[29,43] This enlarges the contact area between the patella and the trochlea and improves stabilization and centralization. This biomechanical behavior is the cornerstone for the selection of the necessary treatment.

7.2.7.1   Physical Examination

The patella is positioned proximal and often also lateral. Proximalization and lateralization are even increased with full contraction of the quadriceps muscle. The mobility of the patella in extension is also increased to medial and lateral indicating the instability. Manual medio-lateral movements of the patella are very loose, documenting the missing osseous stability and also a constitutional laxity. The stability is improved with higher flexion. The improved stability eliminates also the lateralization and normalizes the gliding mechanism of the patella in flexion.

7.2.7.2   Imaging

Radiographs

Different measurements (Insall-Salvati, Blackburne-Peel, Caton-Deschamps ratios) of patellar height on standard sagittal radiographs are in clinical use, all with reference to the tibia.[2,5,13,15,18,31] But each of the established ratios has their own inherent problems. The definition of patella height relies heavily on the ratio used.[11,49] The patellotrochlear index (PTI) using sagittal MRI is a more functional measurement and therefore MRI is recommended.[2,11]

MR Measurement

The PTI is the best modality to depict patella alta (Fig. 7.19).[2,11] The index measures the true articular relationship between

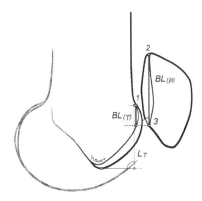

FIGURE 7.19 MR measurement for the patello-trochlear index. *1* Most anterior aspect of the trochlear cartilage, *2* Most superior aspect of the cartilage of the patella, *3* Most inferior aspect of the cartilage of the patella, *BL$_P$* Baseline Patella, *BL$_T$* Baseline trochlea

the patella and the trochlea. Normal values are around 30% (BL$_T$:BL$_P$). Index values of <10% document patella alta.[11]

7.2.7.3   Surgery

Surgical treatment aims to improve the patellofemoral contact and to keep the patella in the trochlea. Excessive proximalization must be corrected. This can be achieved by distalization of the whole extensor apparatus. The amount of distalization is calculated using the PTI. The osteotomy of the tibial tubercle is performed in the horizontal plane with a distal oblique cut. A piece of bone with the calculated length is removed after a second cut. The tibial tubercle is finally fixed with two compression screws. Imbrication or lengthening of the medial or lateral soft tissue structures may be necessary.

7.2.7.4   Postoperative Rehabilitation

Partial weight bearing (15 kg) is recommended for 6 weeks. ROM is slowly increased during the first 6 weeks, maximal to 90° of knee flexion. Straight leg rising is not allowed for 6 weeks. The complete recovery time takes 4 months.

7.3   Tibia

7.3.1   Increased TT/TG

Increased tibial tubercle–trochlear groove (TT-TG) distance is a radiographic measurement tool representing normal or increased lateralization of the tibial tuberosity. Medialization osteotomy of the tibial tubercle has often been performed in patients with patellofemoral complaints and normal TT-TG distance. Hence, tibial tubercle is transposed to a nonanatomic position. We believe that more restricted indication must be made.

7.3.1.1   Physical Examination

The most obvious finding during physical examination is the lateral patellar position in extension. Lateral dynamic patellar subluxation and tilt may occur when the quadriceps muscle is contracted. The Q angle value (measured in extension without muscular contraction) is generally high. A positive patellar apprehension test to lateral may be present. In combination with other pathologies (i.e., trochlear dysplasia), the patella may almost dislocate completely. In isolated disease, the patella typically is well centered in flexion. Also, the tuberculum–sulcus angle (measured in 90° of flexion) is increased (>10° to the lateral).

7.3.1.2   Imaging

Radiographs

The anteroposterior and the lateral view show mild lateral patellar subluxation. Comparative studies of plain x-rays and CT showed that localization of tibial tubercle could not be defined on plain x-rays even with the aid of markers; hence CT is needed.[56]

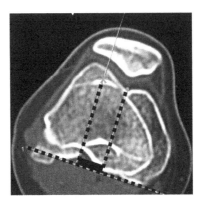

FIGURE 7.20 TT-TG distance measurements on axial CT scans

Axial CT Evaluation

The TT-TG distance is measured on superposed slices of the distal femur and tibial head (Fig. 7.20). First, the epicondylar line is indicated. Second, the anterior part of the tibial tubercle (star) and the trochlear groove (point) are indicated. Then perpendicular lines are drawn to the epicondylar line. The TT-TG distance corresponds to the length between these two lines (thick black line). TT-TG distances of 20 mm and more are considered as pathologic[10] Measurement error on CT-scans has been found around 3.5 mm.[40]

MRI

MRI is of valuable help to depict other patellofemoral pathology and may even measure TT-TG distance.[46,47]

7.3.1.3   Special Considerations

Differential diagnosis of clinical findings of patients with increased TT-TG distance may be vast; however pathologic tuberculum–sulcus angle is pathognomonic. Increased Q angle should not be used alone as indicator for osteotomy of tibial tubercle. Lateralization of the patella, which is found in patients with increased TT-TG distance, typically decreases the Q angle, and the cadaveric trials could not find any correlation between Q angle and patellar instability. Other biases are gynecoid pelvis, genu valgum, and internal foot rotation.

Increased lateralization of the tibial tubercle in extension can be related to the final tibial external rotation with full knee extension.[44] Therefore, tuberculum–sulcus angle is more sensitive.[7]

Concomitant findings, such as patellar dysplasia, constrained lateral retinaculum, and secondary instability due to patellar dislocation have to be taken into consideration when medial transposition of the tibial tubercle is planned, since results after osteotomy are better in lateralized patella than in unstable patellae.[25] In addition, overcorrections may lead to medial patellofemoral and/or even femorotibial medial osteoarthritis.

7.3.1.4   Surgery

Treatment must eliminate the lateral patellar subluxation and tilt. The surgical intervention consists of different steps: Mild medialization of the tibial tubercle in reference to the tubercle–sulcus angle. The tubercle–sulcus angle should be $0°$[38] and the TT-TG distance 10–15 mm. The second step consists of shortening and doubling of the medial soft tissue structures (retinaculum, patellofemoral ligament). The last step is the lengthening of the lateral soft tissue structures; tightness is controlled in extension and flexion (in about $60°$).

The surgical procedure begins with a parapatellar lateral incision and lateral arthrotomy under consideration of the lengthening of the lateral soft tissue structures. The tibial tubercle is partially detached, moved medially, and temporarily fixed with a Kirschner-wire in the planned position (Fig. 7.21). The tubercle–sulcus angle must be controlled in $90°$ of knee flexion. When the tubercle–sulcus angle is $0°$, then the tibial tubercle is fixed definitively with one or two screws. The lateral soft tissue structures are temporarily adapted in $60°$ of knee flexion with some sutures. The position of the patella, the lateral

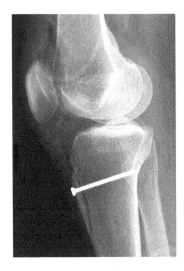

FIGURE 7.21 Screw fixation after medialization of the tibial tubercle

displacement, and the patella glide are then controlled. The patella should remain in the trochlea; the displacement and glide of the patella to medial and lateral should be one to two quadrants.[38] If this is present, no doubling of the medial soft tissue structures is necessary. If the patellar glide or lateral patellar displacement are still pathologic (more than two quadrants), then shortening of the medial patellofemoral ligament in 40° of flexion and the medial retinaculum may be necessary.

7.3.1.5   Postoperative Rehabilitation

First therapeutic aim after surgery is healing of the osteotomy, quadriceps muscle activation, and static and dynamic normalization of the patella balancing in the trochlea. This requests partial weight bearing for 4 weeks with a maximum of 15 kg load and 30 kg until the 7th week after surgery. Straight leg raise is prohibited during this period. Full weight bearing is allowed after healing osteotomy has been confirmed by conventional radiographs. Bicycle and swimming exercises can be initiated 4 weeks after surgery. After 4 months, no restriction in activities is advised.

7.3.1.6   Summary

Medialization of the tibial tubercle has one specific indication: increased TT-TG distance in CT scans (>20 mm) with symptomatic patellar (sub-) dislocation.[10] All different underlying pathologies must be respected for the treatment. Overcorrection of the tibial tubercle to medial must be strictly avoided. Wrong indications for medialization of the tibial tubercle may cause medial patellofemoral and/or femorotibial osteoarthritis.

Anteromedially tubercle transfer can be indicated when lateralization of the patella combined with lateral cartilage destruction is found.[28]

References

1. Albee FH. The bone graft wedge in the treatment of habitual dislocation of the patella.Med Rec. 1915;88:257-9.
2. Barnett AJ, Prentice M, Mandalia V, et al. Patellar height measurement in trochlear dysplasia. Knee Surg Sports Traumatol Arthrosc. 2009;17:1412-5.
3. Bereiter H. Die Trochleaplastik bei Trochleadysplasie zur Therapie der rezidivierenden Patellaluxation. In: Wirth CJ, Rudert M, editors Das Patellofemoral Schmerzsyndrom. Darmstadt: Steinkopff; 2000:162-77.
4. Bereiter H, Gautier E. Die Trochleaplastik als chirurgische Therapie der rezidivierenden Patellaluxation bei Trochleadysplasie des Femurs. Arthroskopie. 1994;7:281-6.
5. Bernageau J, Goutallier D, Debeyre J, et al. Nouvelle technique d'ecploration de l'articulation fémoro-patellaire. Incindinces axiales quadriceps contracté et décontracté.Rev Chir Orthop Reparatrice Appar Mot. 1969;61(suppl 2):286-90.

6. Biedert RM. Is there an indication for lateral release and how I do it. Paper presented at: International Patellofemoral Study Group; 2000; Garmisch-Partenkirchen,Germany.
7. Biedert RM. Patellofemoral disorders: diagnosis and treatment. New York: Wiley; 2000.
8. Biedert RM. Measurements of the length of the proximal and distal trochlea and the trochlear depth on sagittal MRI in patients wieht lateral patellar subluxation. Paper presented at International Patellofemoral Study Group, Lausanne, Switzerland, 2005.
9. Biedert RM. Trochlea dysplasia: indications for trochleoplasty (deepening) and raising/shortening/lengthening of flat/short lateral trochlea. Paper presented at International Patellofemoral Study Group, Boston, 2006.
10. Biedert RM. Osteotomies. Orthopade. 2008;37:872-83.
11. Biedert RM, Albrecht S. The patellotrochlear index: a new index for assessing patellar height. Knee Surg Sports Traumatol Arthrosc. 2006;14:707-12.
12. Biedert RM, Bachmann M. Anterior-posterior trochlear measurements of normal and dysplastic trochlea by axial magnetic resonance imaging. Knee Surg Sports Traumatol Arthrosc. 2009;17:1225-30.
13. Biedert RM, Gruhl C. Axial computed tomography of the patellofemoral joint with and without quadriceps contraction. Arch Orthop Trauma Surg. 1997;116:77-82.
14. Biedert RM, Netzer P, Gal I, et al. The lateral condyle index: a new index for assessing the length of the lateral articular trochlea. Paper presented at International Patellofemoral Study Group, Boston, 2006.
15. Blackburne JS, Peel TE. A new method of measuring patellar height. J Bone Joint Surg. 1977;59-B:241-2.
16. Bruce WD, Stevens PM. Surgical correction of miserable malalignment syndrome. J Pediatr Orthop. 2004;24:392-6.
17. Carrillon Y, Abidi H, Dejour D, et al. Patellar instability: assessment on MR images by measuring the lateral trochlear inclination-initial experience. Radiology. 2000;216:582-5.
18. Caton J, Deschamps G, Chambat P, et al. Patella infera. Apropos of 128 cases. Rev Chir Orthop Reparatrice Appar Mot. 1982;68:317-25.
19. Dejour D, Le Coultre B. Osteotomies in patello-femoral instabilities. Sports Med Arthrosc. 2007;15:39-46.
20. Dejour D, Locatelli E. Patellar instability in adults. Surg Tech Orthop Traumatol. 2001;55:1-6.
21. Dejour H, Walch G, Neyret P, et al. Dysplasia of the femoral trochlea. Rev Chir Orthop Reparatrice Appar Mot. 1990;76:45-54.
22. Dejour H, Walch G, Nove-Josserand L, et al. Factors of patellar instability: an anatomic radiographic study. Knee Surg Sports Traumatol Arthrosc. 1994;2:19-26.

23. Dejour H, Walch G, Nove-Josserand L, et al. Factors of patellar instability: an anatomoradigraphic analysis. In: Feagin JA Jr, editor The curcial ligaments. Diagnosis and treatment of ligament injuries about the knee. New York: Churchill Livingstone; 1994. p. 261-367.

24. Delgado ED, Schoenecker PL, Rich MM, et al. Treatment of severe torsional malalignment syndrome. J Pediatr Orthop. 1996;16:484-8.

25. Diks MJF, Wymenga AB, Anderson PG. Patients with lateral tracking patella have better pain relief following CT-guided tuberosity transfer than patients with unstable patella. Knee Surg Sports Traumatol Arthrosc. 2003;11:384-8.

26. Donell ST, Joseph G, Hing CB, et al. Modified Dejour trochleoplasty for severe dysplasia: operative technique and early clinical results. Knee. 2006;13:266-73.

27. Feinstein WK, Noble PC, Kamaric E, et al. Anatomic alignment of the patellar groove. Clin Orthop Relat Res. 1996;331:64-73.

28. Fulkerson JP, Becker GJ, Meaney JA, et al. Anteromedial tibial tubercle transfer without bone graft. Am J Sports Med. 1990; 18:490-6.

29. Goodfellow J, Hungerford DS, Zindel M. Patello-femoral joint mechanics and pathology. 1. Functional anatomy of the patello-femoral joint. J Bone Joint Surg. 1976;58-B:287-90.

30. Grelsamer RP, Proctor CS, Bazos AN. Evaluation of patellar shape in the sagittal plane. A clinical analysis. Am J Sports Med. 1994; 22:61-6.

31. Grelsamer RP, Tedder JL. The lateral trochlear sign. Femoral trochlear dysplasia as seen on a lateral view roentgenograph. Clin Orthop Relat Res. 1992;281:159-62.

32. Heegaard J, Leyvraz PF, Curnier A, et al. The biomechanics of the human patella during passive knee flexion. J Biomech. 1995;28: 1265-79.

33. Heegaard J, Leyvraz PF, Van Kampen A, et al. Influence of soft structures on patellar three-dimensional tracking. Clin Orthop Relat Res. 1994;299:235-43.

34. Hille E, Schulitz KP, Henrichs C, et al. Pressure and contract-surface measurements within the femoropatellar joint and their variations following lateral release. Arch Orthop Trauma Surg. 1985;104:275-82.

35. Hoppenfeld S, DeBoer P. Surgical exposures in orthopaedics: the anatomic approach. Philadelphia: Lippincott Williams & Wilkins; 2003.

36. Insall J, Salvati E. Patella position in the normal knee joint. Radiology. 1971;101:101-4.

37. James SL, Bates BT, Osternig LR. Injuries to runners. Am J Sports Med. 1978;6:40-50.

38. Kolowich PA, Paulos LE, Rosenberg TD, et al. Lateral release of the patella: indications and contraindications. Am J Sports Med. 1990;18:359-65.

39. Lee TQ, Anzel SH, Bennett KA, et al. The influence of fixed rotational deformities of the femur on the patellofemoral contact pressures in human cadaver knees. Clin Orthop Relat Res. 1994;302:69-74.

40. Lustig S, Servien E, Aït Si Selmi T, et al. Factors affecting reliability of TT-TG measurements before and after medialization: a CT scan study. Rev Chir Orthop Reparatrice Appar Mot. 2007;92:429-36.

41. Malaghem J, Maldague B. Depth insufficiency of the proximal trochlear groove on lateral radiographs of the knee: relation to patellar dislocation. Radiology. 1989;170:507-10.

42. Masse Y. Trochleoplasty. Restoration of the intercondylar groove in subluxations and dislocations of the patella. Rev Chir Orthop Reparatrice Appar Mot. 1978;64:3-17.

43. Müller W, Wirz D. Anatomie, Biomechanik und Dynamik des Patellofemoralgelenks. In: Wirth CJ, Rudert M, editors Das Patellofemorale Schmerzsyndrom. Darmstadt: Steinkopff; 2000. p. 3-19.

44. Pagenstert GI, Bachmann M. Klinische Untersuchung bei patellofemoralen Problemen. Orthopade. 2008;37:890-903.

45. Percy EC, Strother RT. Patellalgia. Physician Sportsmed. 1985;13:43-59.

46. Schoettle PB, Zanetti M, Seifert B, Pfirrmann CW, Fucentese SF, Romero J. The tibial tuberosity-trochlear groove distance: a comparative study between CT and MRI scanning. Knee. 2006;13(1):26-31.

47. Schoettle PB, Zanetti M, Seifert B, et al. The tibial tuberosity-trochlear groove distance; a comparative study between CT and MRI scanning. Knee. 2006;13:26-31.

48. Scuderi GR. Surgical treatment for patellar instability. Orthop Clin North Am. 1992;23:619-30.

49. Seil R, Muller B, Georg T, et al. Reliability and interobserver variability in radiological patellar height ratios. Knee Surg Sports Traumatol Arthrosc. 2000;8:231-6.

50. Servien E, Neyret P, Si Selmi TA, et al. Radiographs. In: Biedert RM, editor Patellofemoral disorders: diagnosis and treatment. New York: Wiley; 2004. p. 87-100.

51. Tecklenburg K, Dejour D, Hoser C, et al. Bony and cartilaginous anatomy of the patellofemoral joint. Knee Surg Sports Traumatol Arthrosc. 2006;14:235-40.

52. van Huyssteen AL, Hendrix MR, Barnett AJ, et al. Cartilage-bone mismatch in the dysplastic trochlea. An MRI study. J Bone Joint Surg. 2006;88-B:688-91.

53. van Kampen A, Huiskes R. The three-dimensional tracking pattern of the human patella. J Orthop Res. 1990;8:372-82.

54. Verdonk R, Jansegers E, Stuyts B. Trochleoplasty in dysplastic knee trochlea. Knee Surg Sports Traumatol Arthrosc. 2005;13:529-33.

55. Von Knoch E, Böhm T, Bürgi ML, et al. Trochleaplasty for recurrent patellar dislocation in association with trochlear dysplasia. J Bone Joint Surg Br. 2006;88-B:1331-5.
56. Wagenaar F, Koeter S, Anderson P, et al. Conventional radiography cannot replace CT scanning in detecting tibial tubercle lateralisation. Knee. 2007;14:51-4.

Chapter 8
Sulcus Deepening Trochleoplasty

David Dejour and Paulo Renato F. Saggin

8.1 Introduction

Trochlear dysplasia is defined as abnormal shape of the trochlea. It can be shallow, flat, or convex (Fig. 8.1). This anatomic status fails to provide adequate constraint to the

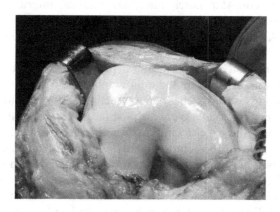

FIGURE 8.1 High-grade trochlear dysplasia (anterior view of a *right* knee). There is no sulcus, and in the lateral aspect (*left*) a big bump can be observed

P.R.F. Saggin (✉)
Instituto de Ortopedia e Traumatologia (I.O.T.),
Passo Fundo, RS, Brazil
e-mail: paulosaggin@yahoo.com.br

V. Sanchis-Alfonso (ed.), *Patellar Instability Surgery in Clinical Practice,* DOI 10.1007/978-1-4471-4501-1_8,
© Springer-Verlag London 2013

normal patellar tracking. Trochlear dysplasia is found in 96% of the population with objective patellar dislocation (at least one true dislocation).[8] This clearly demonstrates its importance in the genesis of the instability. Trochleoplasty is the surgical procedure used to correct trochlear dysplasia. Sulcus deepening trochleoplasty is one of the techniques. It was described by Masse in 1978.[12] Later, Henri Dejour has modified and standardized the procedure.[7]

8.2   Radiologic Features and Classification

X-ray lateral projections of normal trochleae (obtained with perfect superimposition of both femoral condyles) will typically show the contour of the facets, and posterior to them, the line representing the deepest points of the groove.[10,11] The line representing the bottom of the groove is continuous with the intercondylar notch line, and extends anteriorly and proximally. It may end posteriorly to the condyles line (type A) or join the medial condyle line in the superior part of the trochlea (type B).[7]

Trochlear dysplasia, on lateral projections, is defined by the crossing sign, where the radiographic line of the trochlear sulcus crosses (or reaches) the projection of the anterior part of the femoral condyles or trochlear facets. The crossing point represents the exact location where the groove reaches the same height of the femoral condyles, meaning that the trochlea becomes flat in this exact location. The position of the trochlear groove is abnormally prominent in relation to the anterior femoral cortex. While in normal knees it is usually at a mean distance of 0.8 mm posterior to a line tangent to the anterior femoral cortex, in knees with dysplastic trochlea its mean position is 3.2 mm forward this same line[8] (Fig. 8.2).

Two other features are typical of dysplastic trochleae on lateral views: the supratrochlear spur and the double contour sign. The supratrochlear spur can be clearly identified during the surgical exposure, located in the superolateral aspect of the trochlea. It corresponds to an attempt of containing the

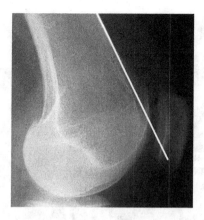

FIGURE 8.2 The trochlear bump is calculated as the amount of trochlea which is in front of a line parallel to the anterior femoral cortex. Alternatively, the sulcus floor position can also be calculated from this line

lateral displacement of the patella. The double contour represents the subchondral bone of the medial hypoplastic facet, seen posterior to the lateral one on this projection (Fig. 8.3). Based on these signs, trochlear dysplasia may be classified in four types (Fig. 8.4)[6,16]:

- Type A: presence of crossing sign on the lateral true view. The trochlea is shallower than normal, but still symmetric and concave.
- Type B: crossing sign and trochlear spur. The trochlea is flat or convex in axial images.
- Type C: there is the presence of the crossing sign and the double-contour sign on the lateral view, representing the densification of the subchondral bone of the medial hypoplastic facet. There is no spur, and in axial views, the lateral facet is convex and the medial hypoplastic.
- Type D: combines all the mentioned signs: crossing sign, supratrochlear spur, and double-contour sign. In axial view, there is clear asymmetry of the facets height, also referred to as a cliff pattern.

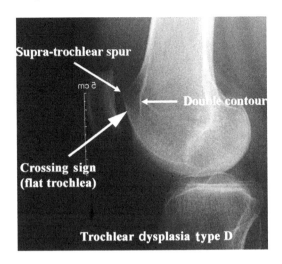

FIGURE 8.3 To analyze the trochlear dysplasia a true profile is needed with a perfect superimposition of the posterior femoral condyles. The three trochlear dysplasia signs are: (1) the crossing sign; (2) the supratrochlear spur; and (3) the double-contour which goes below the crossing sign

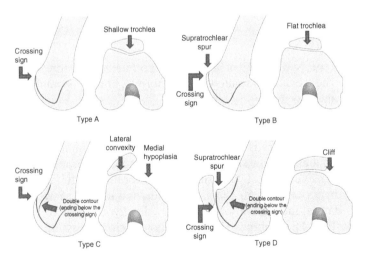

FIGURE 8.4 Trochlear dysplasia classification according to David Dejour

Axial views obtained at 45° (Merchant) will allow the measurement of the sulcus angle.[13] From the point of the bottom of the groove, two lines are drawn connecting it with the most superior point of each facet. The mean normal value defined by Merchant was 138° (SD ± 6), and angles greater than 150° are considered abnormal. Abnormal (dysplastic) trochleae will show higher angles, and at times, no measurement can be made, since there is no sulcus. Alternatively, 30° views will provide those measurements with better trochlear shape assessment.[5] The subjective impression of the trochlear shape is very important, and should be taken in no more than 45° of knee flexion. Greater flexion angles show the lower part of the trochlea, where it becomes deeper, and the examiner can miss the trochlear dysplasia.

The computerized tomography scan will help the x-ray analysis by giving a complete analysis of the trochlea, from the top to the lower part. Tridimensional reconstruction can also be obtained for global shape assessment. Magnetic resonance imaging is another modality in which dysplasia is well documented and the cartilaginous shape of the sulcus can be evaluated.

8.3   Function and Biomechanics

To understand the principles of modifying trochlear shape, its function must be well understood. The lateral facet of the trochlea is oriented obliquely in both sagittal and coronal planes. It deviates anteriorly and laterally from the bottom of the groove. The articulating opposed lateral patellar surface follows this orientation. The patella rests in front of the femoral cortex in total extension, but engages the trochlea in early flexion. A posteriorly directed force, the patellofemoral reaction force, pushes the patella against the trochlea, and as a result of the articulating surfaces orientation, a medial vector is created, directing patellar tracking.[2] The mediolateral tracking of the patella has been shown as highly erratic in cases of trochlear dysplasia.[3]

From this biomechanical explanation, one conclusion is obvious: the trochlea guides patellar tracking. Not only patellar subluxation or lateral displacement is dependent on trochlear shape, but also patellar tilt. There is a high statistical correlation between patellar tilt and the type of trochlear dysplasia.[16] The more severe the dysplasia, the higher the patellar tilt.

Other feature, not included in trochlear function, but derived from the same principle is that patellofemoral reaction force depends on the trochlear prominence. The bigger the trochlear prominence, the greater the compressive reaction force, thus creating an "antimaquet" effect. Inversely, by diminishing the protrusion, the reaction force is also expected to be diminished.

8.4   Goals

Deepening trochleoplasty is proposed to correct trochlear dysplasia, creating a new and more anatomic sulcus and restoring patellar stability. It also corrects the excessive trochlear prominence, thus decreasing the patellofemoral reaction force.

8.5   Indications

Trochleoplasty indications are precise: high-grade trochlear dysplasia with patellar instability and/or abnormal patellar tracking, in the absence of established osteoarthritis. Open growth plates are a contraindication to this type of trochleoplasty. The type of dysplasia should be observed when indicating the procedure, since not all procedures fit all deformities. Types B and D are the most suitable to sulcus deepening trochleoplasty.

Patients with type C dysplasia are not good candidates to the procedure, since there is no prominence to be corrected. They can be submitted to an alternative procedure (lateral facet elevating trochleoplasty), despite the controversy about its long-term results. Type A dysplasia is not suitable to any trochlear procedure. It is also not considered high-grade trochlear dysplasia. Major instability or maltracking, if present, should be attributed to other anatomical abnormalities (excessive tibial tubercle – trochlear groove distance, excessive patellar tilt, or patella alta).

The degree of instability should also be taken into account. Trochleoplasty, as any other surgical procedure, is liable to failure, and this should be considered when indicating the procedure to a patient with mild symptoms, and when no conservative treatment has been proposed yet.

As important as a precise indication, the evaluation and correction of associated abnormalities have to be accomplished (tibial tubercle–trochlear groove distance, patella alta, and patellar tilt). TT-TG correction is not always necessary as the trochleoplasty procedure lateralizes the groove, thus diminishing the TT-TG distance. The sulcus deepening trochleoplasty should be understood as part of the *menu à la carte* (specific procedures for each of the main factors in patellar instability). We routinely associate a soft tissue procedure to the trochleoplasty. Formerly, a VMO plasty was added. Since 2003 medial patellofemoral ligament (MPFL) reconstruction is the procedure of choice.

8.6   Surgical Technique

The procedure is performed under regional anesthesia, complemented with patient sedation. The patient is positioned supine. The entire extremity is prepared and draped, and incision is performed with the extremity flexed by 90°. A straight midline skin incision is carried out from the superior patellar margin until the tibiofemoral articulation. The extremity is then positioned in extension and a medial full thickness skin flap is developed. The arthrotomy is performed through a midvastus adapted approach: medial retinaculum sharp dissection starting over the 1–2 cm medial border of the patella, and blunt dissection of VMO fibers starting distally, at

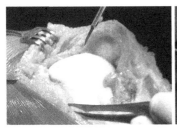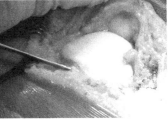

FIGURE 8.5 Surgical exposure. The periosteum is incised along the osteochondral edge and reflected away from the trochlear margin. The anterior femoral cortex should be visible to guide the bone resection

the superomedial pole of the patella, extending approximately 4 cm into the muscle belly.

The patella is not everted but a careful inspection of chondral injuries using ICRS classification and proper treatment (flap resection, microfracture, autologous chondrocyte implantation) is done if requested, and then the patella is retracted laterally. The trochlea is exposed and peritrochlear synovium and periosteum are incised along their osteochondral junction, and reflected from the field using a periosteal elevator (Fig. 8.5). The anterior femoral cortex should be visible to orientate the amount of deepening. Changing the degree of flexion-extension of the knee allows a better view of the complete operatory field and avoids extending the incision.

Once the trochlea is fully exposed, the new one is planned and drawn with a sterile pen. The new trochlear groove is drawn using as starting point the intercondylar notch. From there, a straight line representing it is directed proximally and 3–6° laterally. The superior limit is the osteochondral edge. Two divergent lines are also drawn, starting at the notch and going proximally through the condylotrochlear grooves, representing the lateral and the medial facet limits. They should not enter the tibiofemoral articulation (Fig. 8.6).

The next step is accessing the under surface of the femoral trochlea. For this purpose, a thin strip of cortical bone is removed all around the trochlea. The width of the strip is equal

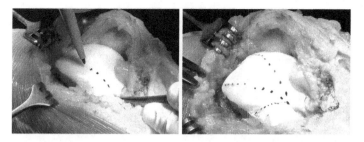

FIGURE 8.6 After the surgical exposure, the new trochlea is drawn. From the intercondylar notch, the bottom of the sulcus and the facets are planned

to the prominence of the trochlea from the anterior femoral cortex, i.e., the bump formed. A sharp osteotome is used and gently tapped. A rongeur is used next, to remove the bone.

Subsequently, cancellous bone must be removed from the under surface of the trochlea. A drill with a depth guide set at 5 mm is used to ensure uniform thickness of the osteochondral flap, thus maintaining an adequate amount of bone attached to the cartilage. The guide also avoids injuring the cartilage or getting too close to it; otherwise thermal injury could be produced. The shell produced must be sufficiently compliant to allow modeling without being fractured. Cancellous bone removal is extended until the notch. More bone is removed from the central portion where the new trochlear groove will rest.

Light pressure should be able to model the flap to the underlying cancellous bone bed in the distal femur. The groove, and sometimes the lateral facet external margin, should be cut to allow further modeling, which is done by gently tapping over a scalpel (Fig. 8.7). If the correction obtained is satisfactory, the new trochlea is fixed with two staples (K-Wires of one millimeter diameter modeled upon the trochlear shape), one in each side of the groove. The staples are fixed with one arm in the cartilaginous upper part of each facet and the other arm in the anterior femoral cortex (Fig. 8.8). Patellar tracking is tested and measures may be obtained. Periosteum and synovial tissue are sutured to the osteochondral edge and anchored to the staples.

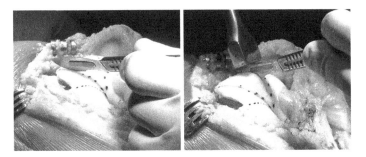

FIGURE 8.7 In order to allow further modeling to the underlying bone bed, the osteochondral flaps may be cut in the sulcus and facets lines

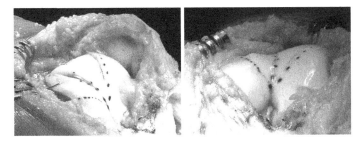

FIGURE 8.8 Lateral and anterior views of dysplastic trochlea after trochleoplasty. Notice that the sulcus and facets relationship resembles a "normal trochlea"

8.7 Postoperative Care

Trochleoplasty does not need weight protection or range of motion limitation. Movement like CPM (continuous passive motion) may also improve cartilage healing. Quadriceps wasting is another negative outcome of immobilization. The main principles guiding trochleoplasty rehabilitation are presented here, but the associated procedures performed have to be taken into account, and rehabilitation has to fit them too.

The rehabilitation is divided in three phases and specific goals depend on the phase. Phase 1 starts the day after the surgery and ends at the 45th day. Passive and active range of motion is encouraged to improve the nutrition of the cartilage and to allow further modeling of the trochlea by patellar tracking. Immediate weight bearing is allowed (with crutches and an extension brace for 4 weeks). Walking without the brace is allowed generally after 1 month depending on the quadriceps recovery. Range of motion is gradually regained (avoiding forced or painful postures). Dynamic quadriceps strengthening with weights on the feet or tibial tubercle is prohibited; only isometric contraction and stimulation are allowed.

Phase 2 goes from the 46th day until the 90th day. Cycling is possible with weak resistance initially. Active ascension of the patella can be performed seated, with the leg stretched and the knee unlocked, by static and isometric quadriceps contractions. Active exercises are added but dynamic and isometric quadriceps strengthening with weights on the feet or tibial tubercle is still forbidden. The anterior and posterior muscular chains are stretched. Weight-bearing proprioception exercises are started when full extension is complete, first in bipodal stance and later in monopodal stance when there is no pain.

Phase 3 is passed from the fourth until the sixth month: this is the sports phase. Running can be initiated on a straight line. Closed kinetic chain muscular reinforcement between 0° and 60° with minor loads but long series are allowed. Stretching of the anterior and posterior muscular chains is continued. The patient is encouraged to proceed with the rehabilitation on his own. After 6 months sports on a recreational or competitive level can be resumed.

Six weeks postoperatively control radiographs, including AP and lateral views (Fig. 8.9) and an axial view in 30° of flexion, are taken. After 6 months a control CT scan is performed in order to document the obtained correction (Fig. 8.10).

8.8   Results

Two series reviewing deepening trochleoplasty were published in the *10èmes Journées Lyonnaises de Chirurgie du Genou* in 2002:

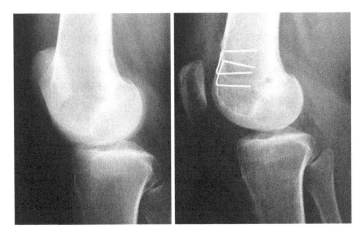

FIGURE 8.9 Pre- and postoperative lateral x-rays showing the resection of the supratrochlear bump and trochlear prominence correction. Additionally, patellar tilt is clearly improved

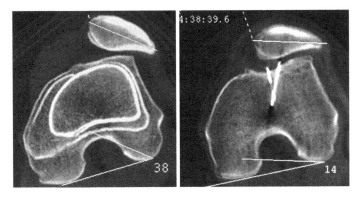

FIGURE 8.10 CT scan axial views before and after trochleoplasty. The trochlear sulcus is restored and patellar tilt is corrected. Patellar subluxation is also improved

The first group included 18 patients, who failed patellar surgery for instability. The mean age at surgery was 24 years. There were no patients lost to follow-up. The mean follow-up was 6 years (2–8 years). The new surgery was six times indicated for pain and 12 times for recurrence of instability. The average number of surgeries before the trochleoplasty was two. The deepening trochleoplasty was associated to a tibial tubercle medialization in eight patients, in six to a tibial tubercle distalization, and all to a VMO plasty. All patients were reviewed clinically with the IKDC form and radiographically. Sixty five percent were satisfied or very satisfied. The knee stability was rated 13 times A and five times B. Twenty eight percent of the patients had residual pain, and this was correlated to the cartilage status at surgery. Two patients developed patellofemoral arthritis. The mean patellar tilt was 35° (18–48°) in the preoperative setting, and improved to 21°(11–28°) with the quadriceps relaxed and 24° (16–32°) with the quadriceps contracted after the surgery.

In the second group there were 44 patients. They had no antecedents of patellofemoral surgery. The mean follow-up was 7 years (2–9 years). Twenty-two tibial tubercle medializations, 26 distalizations, and 32 VMO plasties were associated at the time of surgery. These patients were also reviewed clinically with the IKDC form and radiographically. Eighty five percent were satisfied or very satisfied. The knee stability was rated 31 times A and 13 times B. Five percent had residual pain, but this was not correlated to the cartilage status at surgery. No patellofemoral arthritis was noted. The mean patellar tilt preoperatively was 33° (24–52°), and improved postoperatively to 18° (9°–30°) with the quadriceps relaxed and 22° (14–34°) with the quadriceps contracted.

Verdonk et al.[17] described 13 procedures (deepening trochleoplasty) with a mean follow-up of 18 months. Patients were assessed using the Larsen–Lauridsen score considering pain, stiffness, patellar crepitus, flexion, and loss of function. Seven patients scored poorly, three fairly, and three well. On a subjective scoring system, however, six patients rated the result as very good, four as good, and one as satisfactory. Only two patients found the result inadequate and would never undergo the procedure again. Thus, 77% were satisfied with the procedure.

Donnel et al.[9] described 15 patients (17 knees) submitted to deepening trochleoplasty with a mean follow-up of 3 years. Trochleoplasty was indicated if there was a boss greater than 6 mm, and associated procedures were performed as required. Of the 17 knees, 9 had undergone previous surgery for patellar instability. The boss height was reduced, postoperatively, from an average of 7.5 to 0.7 mm. Tracking became normal in 11 knees and 6 had a slight J-sign. Seven knees had mild residual apprehension. Seven patients were very satisfied, six were satisfied, and two were disappointed. The Kujala score improved from an average of 48 to 75 out of 100.

A different procedure (Bereiter's trochleoplasty[4]) has also been documented in two series by von Knoch et al.[18] and Schottle et al.[14] with good results.

8.9   Complications

Patients submitted to trochleoplasty are at risk for the same complications inherent to any surgical procedure – infection, deep venous thrombosis, etc. Specific complications include trochlear necrosis, incongruence with the patella, hypo- or hypercorrection, and cartilage damage. Schottle performed biopsies in three patients after trochleoplasty, showing cartilage cell viability and flap healing. He concluded that the risk of cartilage damage is low.[15]

Incongruence with the patella is another concern. Studies with longer follow-ups are needed before any assumptions can be made about its consequences. Also, arthritis development is multifactorial, and all patients operated on for patellofemoral instability seem more prone to degeneration than those treated conservatively.

Arthrofibrosis incidence varies between series, but is always a possibility in patellofemoral surgery. Verdonk et al.[17] reported 5 cases in 13 patients, while von Knoch et al.[18] reported that all patients had full range of motion in the final visit. The number of previous or associated procedures is variable, and this can interfere with data interpretation.

Recurrence of instability is very rare after such procedure, and is more likely to result from missed associated abnormalities. The procedure results for pain are not consistent, and although it seems to improve it, some patients may complain of worsening.

8.10   Alternative Procedures

8.10.1   Lateral Facet Elevating Trochleoplasty

This procedure was pioneered by Albee in 1915.[1] It consists of an oblique osteotomy under the lateral facet, where a corticocancellous bone wedge is interposed, with the apex medial and the base lateral. The osteotomy advances until the place of the trochlear groove, but does not disrupt it, producing a hinge in its medial aspect. The result is that it elevates the more lateral aspect of the trochlear lateral facet, and also increases its obliquity, thus increasing the containment force acting on the patella. At least 5 mm of subchondral bone should be maintained to avoid trochlear necrosis.

It is effective for patellar containment, but at the same time it increases the patellofemoral reaction force when it increases the trochlear protuberance. Pain and arthritis may result from this.

8.10.2   Bereiter Trochleoplasty

This technique was described by Bereiter and Gautier in 1994.[4] In this method, a lateral parapatellar approach is performed, the trochlea exposed, and the synovium dissected away from it. Then, a thin osteochondral flake with 2 mm of subchondral bone is elevated from the trochlea extending until the intercondylar notch. The distal femoral subchondral bone is deepened and refashioned with osteotomes and a high-speed burr. Next, the osteochondral flap is seated in the refashioned bed, and fixed with 3 mm wide vicryl bands, passing through the center of the groove and exiting in the lateral femoral condyle. The periosteum is reattached to the edge of the cartilage and closure of the wound is performed.

8.11   Conclusion

Deepening trochleoplasty is a very rare procedure in the objective patellar dislocation group. It concerns only patients with high-grade trochlear dysplasia types B or D and abnormal patellar tracking. It is part of the "menu à la carte" which leads to the correction of the anatomical abnormalities, one by one. The technical procedure is highly demanding and prone to complications. It is, however, very effective in providing stability.

References

1. Albee F. Bone graft wedge in the treatment of habitual dislocation of the patella. Med Rec. 1915;88:257-9.
2. Amis AA. Current concepts on anatomy and biomechanics of patellar stability. Sports Med Arthrosc. 2007;15:48-56.
3. Amis AA, Oguz C, Bull AM, et al. The effect of trochleoplasty on patellar stability and kinematics: a biomechanical study in vitro. J Bone Joint Surg. 2008;90-B:864-9.
4. Bereiter H, Gautier E. Die trochleaplastik als chirurgische therapie der rezidivierenden patellaluxation bei trochleadysplasie des femurs. Arthroskopie. 1994;7:281-6.
5. Davies AP, Bayer J, Owen-Johnson S, et al. The optimum knee flexion angle for skyline radiography is thirty degrees. Clin Orthop Relat Res. 2004;423:166-71.
6. Dejour D, Le Coultre B. Osteotomies in patello-femoral instabilities. Sports Med Arthrosc. 2007;15:39-46.
7. Dejour H, Walch G, Neyret P, et al. Dysplasia of the femoral trochlea. Rev Chir Orthop Reparatrice Appar Mot. 1990;76:45-54.
8. Dejour H, Walch G, Nove-Josserand L, et al. Factors of patellar instability: an anatomic radiographic study. Knee Surg Sports Traumatol Arthrosc. 1994;2:19-26.

9. Donell ST, Joseph G, Hing CB, et al. Modified Dejour trochleoplasty for severe dysplasia: operative technique and early clinical results. Knee. 2006;13:266-73.

10. Maldague B, Malghem J. Significance of the radiograph of the knee profile in the detection of patellar instability. Preliminary report. Rev Chir Orthop Reparatrice Appar Mot. 1985;71(suppl 2):5-13.

11. Malghem J, Maldague B. Depth insufficiency of the proximal trochlear groove on lateral radiographs of the knee: relation to patellar dislocation. Radiology. 1989;170:507-10.

12. Masse Y. Trochleoplasty. Restoration of the intercondylar groove in subluxations and dislocations of the patella. Rev Chir Orthop Reparatrice Appar Mot. 1978;64:3-17.

13. Merchant AC, Mercer RL, Jacobsen RH, et al. Roentgenographic analysis of patellofemoral congruence. J Bone Joint Surg. 1974; 56-A:1391-6.

14. Schottle PB, Fucentese SF, Pfirrmann C, et al. Trochleaplasty for patellar instability due to trochlear dysplasia: a minimum 2-year clinical and radiological follow-up of 19 knees. Acta Orthop. 2005;76:693-8.

15. Schottle PB, Schell H, Duda G, et al. Cartilage viability after tro- chleoplasty. Knee Surg Sports Traumatol Arthrosc. 2007;15:161-7.

16. Tavernier T, Dejour D. Knee imaging: what is the best modality. J Radiol. 2001;82:387-405; 407-8.

17. Verdonk R, Jansegers E, Stuyts B. Trochleoplasty in dysplastic knee trochlea. Knee Surg Sports Traumatol Arthrosc. 2005;13:529-33.

18. von Knoch F, Bohm T, Burgi ML, et al. Trochleaplasty for recurrent patellar dislocation in association with trochlear dysplasia. A 4 to 14-year follow-up study. J Bone Joint Surg. 2006;88-B:1331-5.

Index

V. Sanchis-Alfonso (ed.), *Patellar Instability Surgery
in Clinical Practice,* DOI 10.1007/978-1-4471-4501-1,
© Springer-Verlag London 2013